MW01241463

Enlightening, Adjusting and Savings Lives

10

Tenth Edition

Over 20 Years of Real-Life Stories from People Who Turned to Us for Answers

(Updated with Even More New Stories)

By
Dr. Paul Baker, Dr. Patrick Baker and Hundreds of Patients

www.bakerchiropractic.org

By Dr. Paul Baker, Dr. Patrick Baker and Hundreds of Patients

Foreword

In early 2012, we published the first edition of this book. It has become an extremely helpful tool for people who are considering our chiropractic care. We have received many compliments for publishing a book that simply allows people of all ages and all walks of life to share their stories.

We continue to receive many new testimonials from patients each month as well as updates from patients whose stories continue to develop. In 2013, 2014, 2015, and 2016 we published the 2nd, 3rd, 4th, 5th, 6th, 7th, 8th and 9th editions of this book that incorporated all these new stories and updates. Now, we are publishing this 10th edition which contains a wealth of new and inspiring stories submitted by our patients. We hope these latest real-life stories continue to inspire people and help them recognize the many benefits of our chiropractic care.

Being twin brothers, there are a lot of things in life we have endured together. When we were young boys, health problems hampered the both of us. Dr. Patrick was plagued by asthma and Dr. Paul suffered from gastrointestinal problems. With traditional medical care failing to provide a resolution and determined to help, our dad took us to a cousin who was a chiropractor in Akron, Ohio. Under his care, we were correctly diagnosed and treated with a series of chiropractic adjustments. Dr. Patrick's asthma was resolved and Dr. Paul's severe stomach pains were stopped.

From that point on, we both became fascinated and focused on becoming chiropractors and filling our lives with health. Through our high school and college years, we studied and practiced the essential elements of nutrition and exercise. We encouraged and challenged each other to adopt and incorporate the principles of health and wellness into our everyday lives. These principles are firmly engrained in who we are and why we both chose to become chiropractic physicians.

Over the past 20+ years, we have been fortunate to help people with all types of pain, injury, disorder, and disease. They often times came to us out of desperation and hope. They had followed medical advice, taken prescription medications, or even undergone surgery only to realize their problem wasn't getting any better. Many times, it only got worse.

While we were introduced to chiropractic care over 35 years ago and have been practicing physicians for more than 20 years, it still amazes us how many people either are still not aware of the vital role chiropractic care can have in someone's life or are skeptical of its effectiveness given that it does not rely on the use of pills, injections or surgery.

As you read this book, you will see how many of our patients came to us unsure or skeptical of chiropractic care and quickly realized how we could not only resolve their pain, but change the quality of their life. Our actions always speak louder than our words.

We firmly believe that everyone should reap the many benefits of chiropractic care in order to lead healthy lives enriched with wellness and filled with happiness. However, we understand that people remain skeptical. That's why we feel it's important for someone to read this book and learn why chiropractic care can help remedy many health problems.

The book doesn't contain our thoughts or our opinions. It contains the unedited words of people who had serious health problems and desperately needed answers and help.

In the pages that follow, you will see how a lot of our patients describe their first visit to one of our chiropractic clinics as "skeptical." As they tell their story, you will notice how they gained confidence in our care simply by experiencing positive results. Skepticism quickly subsides when you are open to learning and experiencing first hand.

Throughout the many stories, you will also see how patients came to us for a specific reason and the care we provided resolved not only that health condition, but many others as well.

The best testament of all to our chiropractic care is how our patients refer family members, friends and co-workers to our clinics to relieve them of their pain and health problems.

The skepticism and misunderstanding that still exist are the motivations for this book and why it is presented in this format. We didn't want the reader to study our words. We want to present the reader with the stories of people from all walks of life and have them tell their story of why they took a step towards chiropractic care for help with all sorts of pain, injuries, disorders or disease and how they came to understand the power of the human body when its full potential is unlocked by this type of care.

With knowledge and education comes logical understanding.

If you understand how and why chiropractic care is effective in treating health conditions, it will allow you to see why it can be a vital part of your future and the quality of your life.

We hope the various stories contained within this book may restore hope and promise if you or a loved one is battling a health problem. We also hope it inspires you to look at chiropractic care for answers. It truly is a safe, proven and powerful form of health care.

To learn more about our chiropractic care, please visit **www. bakerchiropractic.org.**

To learn more about us, we invite you to visit **www.doctorspaulandpatrick.com.**

Yours Truly In Health and Wellness,

Dr. Paul Baker and Dr. Patrick Baker

P.S. As you read each chapter of this book, you will see some stories that have been repeated from previous chapters. Because chiropractic care addresses overall health, it is effective in resolving multiple health conditions. Therefore, if a patient was experiencing several health problems, we repeated their story for each of their health conditions.

Baker Chiropractic and Wellness Clinic Locations

1. **Cincinnati – Red Bank**

   4781 Red Bank Rd.
   Cincinnati, Ohio 45227

   Telephone: (513) 561-2273

2. **West Chester**

   7556 Voice of America Centre Dr.
   West Chester, Ohio 45069

   Telephone: (513) 759-4666

3. **Fairfield**

   675 Deis Drive
   Fairfield, Ohio 45014

   Telephone: (513) 858-6700

Some of the <u>visceral</u> conditions chiropractic/ manual therapy may be helpful for

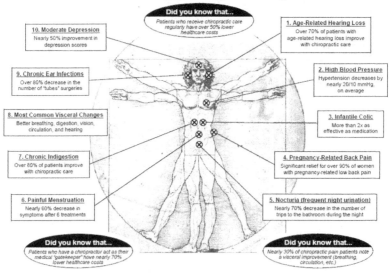

Did you know that...
Patients who receive chiropractic care regularly have over 50% lower healthcare costs

10. Moderate Depression
Nearly 50% improvement in depression scores

1. Age-Related Hearing Loss
Over 70% of patients with age-related hearing loss improve with chiropractic care

9. Chronic Ear Infections
Over 80% decrease in the number of "tubes" surgeries

2. High Blood Pressure
Hypertension decreases by nearly 20/10 mmHg, on average

8. Most Common Visceral Changes
Better breathing, digestion, vision, circulation, and hearing

3. Infantile Colic
More than 2x as effective as medication

7. Chronic Indigestion
Over 80% of patients improve with chiropractic care

4. Pregnancy-Related Back Pain
Significant relief for over 90% of women with pregnancy-related low back pain

6. Painful Menstruation
Nearly 60% decrease in symptoms after 6 treatments

5. Nocturia (frequent night urination)
Nearly 70% decrease in the number of trips to the bathroom during the night

Did you know that...
Patients who have a chiropractor act as their medical "gatekeeper" have nearly 70% lower healthcare costs

Did you know that...
Nearly 30% of chiropractic pain patients note a visceral improvement (breathing, circulation, etc.)

Some of the <u>painful</u> conditions chiropractic/ manual therapy may be helpful for

Did you know that...
Patients, on average, rate their overall satisfaction with chiropractic care as "excellent"

10. Chronic Headache Pain
Over 70% effective for migraine & cervicogenic headaches

1. Chronic Pain in the Neck
Nearly 75% of chronic neck pain patients improve significantly with chiropractic care

9. Pain in the Shoulder
More than 2x as effective as medical care

2. Tennis Elbow Pain
Over 50% of patients note immediate improvement after one treatment

8. Patients with Chronic Arthritis
Over 70% of chronic arthritis patients who have tried chiropractic care think it is effective

3. Carpal Tunnel Syndrome
Almost 70% relief within 3 weeks, on average

7. Chronic Knee Pain
Nearly 50% relief after just 1 treatment, on average

4. Conditions Involving Low Back Pain
Nearly 50% respond significantly within 2 treatments, with an average improvement of 73%

6. Pain in the Ankle
Nearly 40% relief after 1 treatment, on average

5. Leg Pain Due to Herniated Disc
More than 2x as effective as physical therapy

Did you know that...
Over 80% of chiropractic patients are referred by other patients, friends, relatives, etc.

Did you know that...
Over 95% of chiropractic patients would refer a friend or family member for chiropractic care

By Dr. Paul Baker, Dr. Patrick Baker and Hundreds of Patients

"There is more to your spine and central nervous system than people realize. When your spine is out of alignment, it affects your body's health and functioning.

Do yourself a favor and go to Dr. Baker's office and find out what condition your spine is in and what can be done to give yourself one of the greatest benefits to your health and well-being.

Please pass this book on so others can be educated on the benefits of chiropractic care. I highly suggest you go to these doctors because I know first-hand they know what they are doing!

They will teach you and show what a lot of people aren't aware of about spinal correction."

Elizabeth Pinedo

By Dr. Paul Baker, Dr. Patrick Baker and Hundreds of Patients

Contents

By Dr. Paul Baker, Dr. Patrick Baker and Hundreds of Patients

1

Corrective Chiropractic Care

Many chiropractors choose to limit their practice to pain relief only. Getting a patient out of pain without using prescription drugs or surgery is very important.

At Baker Chiropractic and Wellness, we are not just focused on relieving pain. We are also concerned with providing our patients with a future life of health and wellness.

Research shows that when your spine and central nervous system are not in their proper position, they will degenerate silently. This allows organs to malfunction and become susceptible to disease. We want to make sure that doesn't happen.

We practice a type of chiropractic care known as Corrective Care Chiropractic. This form of care is aimed at keeping patients pain-free while also removing any and all interferences with the Central Nervous System. These interferences are called subluxation.

Corrective Care Chiropractic is conducted through a very specific and customized program of spinal adjustments, stretches and exercises that are unique for each patient.

The frequency of the Corrective Care Chiropractic is determined by the severity of subluxation and the position of a patient's spine. Once subluxations have been reduced and normal alignment of the spine has been restored, a patient moves into a less-frequent maintenance program to make sure they are staying subluxation-free and their spine is properly aligned.

As you read the many stories provided by our patients in this book, note how they first came to Baker Chiropractic for pain relief. Once they escaped their pain, they stayed for a life of health and wellness. That's what Corrective Chiropractic Care is all about.

Whether you are living with pain now or not, we invite and encourage you to contact us and experience the many benefits our Corrective Chiropractic Care will provide you. Your future health and quality of life depend on the decisions you make today.

Here's an example of our care from a 68 year-old female patient.

As shown in the below x-ray image, her cervical curve was restored to the ideal 43 degree curvature with Corrective Chiropractic Care at Baker Chiropractic and Wellness.

This patient's hearing was restored as a result of the corrective care.

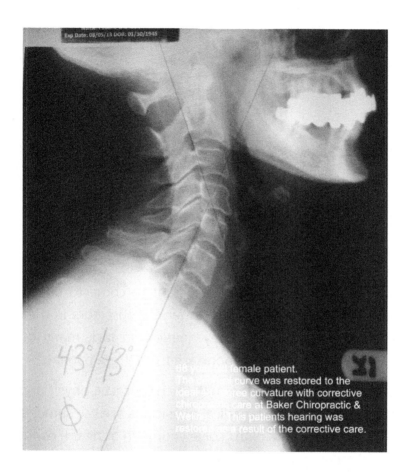

Exp Date: 08/05/13 DOB: 01/30/1945

43°/43°

68 year old female patient.
The [...] curve was restored to the
ideal [...] degree curvature with corrective
chiropractic care at Baker Chiropractic &
Wellness. This patients hearing was
restored as a result of the corrective care.

2
Not All
Chiropractors Are
Created Equal

Some of our patients were reluctant to come to us initially because they had tried going to other chiropractors in the past without getting the results they needed. In fact, many of the stories contained within this book are from these patients.

It's important to know that not all chiropractic physicians are the same, just like not all medical physicians are the same. If the care you were provided didn't solve your pain or health condition and didn't meet your expectations, please don't give up.

Our approach to chiropractic care and our extensive experience enables us to provide our patients with positive results that other chiropractors may not be able to deliver.

We are continually educating and training both ourselves and our staff. Decades of experience, continuing education and routine training provide our patients with the highest level of chiropractic care available. It also provides them with positive results when others fall short.

If you have tried chiropractic care in the past and didn't see the results you expected, please contact us. We are confident we will help you like we have helped so many others.

3
Chiropractic Care During Pregnancy

I decided to get chiropractic work done because I am on my third pregnancy and had a lot of back pain and hip pain. It was incredibly uncomfortable and my acid reflux was awful.

I've only been here now about 4 visits, and I am feeling absolutely no back pain or hip pain! My acid reflux has diminished quite a bit too and now pains that I didn't even realize were there are diminishing as well!

I'm feeling a lot better, my sleep is no longer disrupted, and my mood towards my family is better. I can move around better, and I am not "waddling" as much. I am walking more.

By Dr. Paul Baker, Dr. Patrick Baker and Hundreds of Patients

Thank you Dr. Mike and Baker Chiropractic!

— **Mandy T.**

· · · · ·

Pregnancy is a special time in a woman's life. It's filled with a great joy and anticipation that only a mother knows.

Pregnancy is also a period of dramatic change for a mother's body. Some women easily adapt to the emotional and physical changes associated with pregnancy, while others suffer pain, discomfort and anxiety.

So what steps can a woman take to make her pregnancy a pleasant experience for both her and her baby? Incorporate our chiropractic care before, during and after your pregnancy!

We've played an integral part in the health care of pregnant women and their unborn children for over 20 years.

Here are Three (3) Steps to our prenatal care:

Step 1: Spine and Nervous System

During pregnancy, expectant mothers undergo many physical changes within their bodies in preparation for carrying a child and giving birth. The spine is one of the primary areas where these changes are felt the most and where a majority of problems start as subluxations.

As chiropractors, we are specially trained physicians who keep the spine and nervous system healthy and free from subluxations. Most people don't realize how the spine and nervous system control all parts of the human body. But your developing unborn child certainly does.

When a mother's egg is fertilized and pregnancy begins, cells start to multiple and divide. The first things these cells create are the brain and spinal cord. From the spinal cord, little branches of nerves begin to spread outward. The combination of the brain, spinal cord and nerves becomes the central nervous system. Once the central nervous system is in place, "buds" will form at the end of nerves. These buds are the beginning of all the vital organs such as the heart, liver and kidneys.

The brain and central nervous system literally are the origin of life and control every cell within the body. These cells form tissue, tissue forms organs and organs form systems. Put all these systems together and a human body is created.

The human brain controls every microscopic cell within the body and the brain communicates with each of the millions of cells via the nervous system. This is how the brain delivers the necessary energy and instructions to every part of your body to make it function.

There are many situations where the energy sent by your brain through your nervous system becomes filtered and distorted. This interference is known as a subluxation.

Bones or joints may become misaligned and nerves can become irritated, pinched, stretched or compressed which all causes inference in the flow of energy from the brain. When this energy is distorted or blocked, a variety of symptoms will surface including pain.

As a baby starts to develop and continues to grow, an expectant mother is experiencing 9 months of increasing stress on her bones, muscles and joints which can create subluxations.

We keep mother's-to-be free from subluxations and the pain and discomfort that are caused by these subluxations.

Routine chiropractic care with us can help prevent such common health conditions experienced during pregnancy as:

- Back Aches / Back Pain
- Indigestion
- Insomnia
- Constipation

Step 2: Nutrition and Diet

As outlined above, a healthy spine and nervous system are essential elements of a pleasant, problem-free pregnancy. Another crucial part is proper diet and nutrition.

A mother and her unborn child are dependent upon receiving the correct nutrition for proper development. What mom chooses to eat during pregnancy has an impact on her child receiving the correct nutrition.

We provide our expectant mothers who are patients with important guidance on diet and nutrition during pregnancy so they can make the right food choices for themselves and their baby.

Step 3: Exercise

The third step to a pleasant pregnancy is getting the correct amount of exercise. We work with expectant mothers to develop a customized exercise program that keeps them fit, prepares them for birth and helps them continue to look great after giving birth.

Preparation for Birth

The combination of Steps 1, 2 and 3 outlined above are all elements of our comprehensive chiropractic care that provide numerous benefits to expectant mothers and increase their probability of having an enjoyable pregnancy. The advantages of following our chiropractic care during pregnancy culminate at the birth of the child.

Certain chiropractic techniques relieve stress on the pelvis and uterus which helps the unborn child properly turn and position for a healthy and natural birth.

Webster Technique for Breech Births

Dr. Larry Webster, a chiropractor and founder of the International Chiropractic Pediatric Association developed the Webster Technique as a safe means to restore proper pelvic balance and function. It was developed to restore normal function of the mother and improve her comfort throughout pregnancy in preparation for a safer, easier birth.

Dr. Webster reported that in women who presented with a breech baby, the results of the adjustment appeared to normalize pelvic biomechanics and facilitate optimal fetal positioning. As Dr. Webster taught other doctors of chiropractic this adjustment, they too reported positive changes in baby positioning.

We have been utilizing the Webster Technique throughout our

20+ year history and have seen the benefits of this technique for preventing breech births and facilitating safe and easy births for our patients.

We can help you experience a healthy, safe and enjoyable pregnancy too!

4
Chiropractic Care for Infants and Babies

Forcing, pulling and twisting a baby during birth are very common procedures and may cause subluxations in newborns.

Both natural child birth and C-Sections can be a traumatic experience for a baby. Pulling, twisting and turning are commonly performed during a child's birth. This process will often times create problems in an infant's delicate neck and back resulting in misalignments of the spine and subluxations (interferences) in the infant's central nervous system.

The pinching and irritation of nerves from subluxations derived at birth can lead to a variety of health issues in babies including such ailments as:

1. Colic
2. Fussiness and Irritability
3. Feeding Problems
4. Constipation
5. Sleep Irregularity
6. Breathing Problems

You will find testimonials from mothers in this book about how their children were suffering from conditions like the ones listed above. Moms and dads come to us routinely with babies who are colicky or fussy. Not only is baby uncomfortable, mom and dad are stressed-out from lack of sleep and feeling helpless. In most cases, a subluxation is causing the infant's problems. When we remove the subluxations, the problem gets resolved and everyone – mom, dad and baby – are all happy.

An infant's health may be impaired from his or her first breath when there are problems with the child's nervous system. These problems may show themselves immediately or they may appear years later.

If left undiagnosed and untreated, subluxations can also lead to long term issues as the child grows older including:

1. Headaches
2. Vision Problems
3. Hearing Problems
4. Immune System Deficiencies
5. Learning Disorders

We routinely perform examinations on infants and babies to check for subluxations. When necessary, we also perform very gentle and safe adjustments to remove subluxations that are preventing optimum health.

As a new parent, you want to give your child the best of everything and a future life filled with health and happiness. That's what our Baker Chiropractic and Wellness Lifestyle of Maximized Living is all about.

We aren't just focused on keeping your infant's spine and nervous system in peak condition; we are dedicated to providing your infant with the 5 Essentials for a healthy and fulfilling life, free from diseases, free from disorders and free from reliance on prescription medications.

5
Chiropractic Care for Toddlers

A toddler's body is developing at a very fast pace. In fact by the age of 5 years old, a toddler's spine will have more than doubled in length from birth.

A toddler is subjected to a variety of everyday stresses and traumas that can cause subluxation. Just think how many times a toddler is picked up, carried in different positions and put down. These subtle acts alone could cause subluxation.

As any mother or father knows, toddlers are highly inquisitive and exploratory. Just turn away from them for a minute and they could be anywhere. This curious behavior also causes them to suffer falls, accidental bumps on the head and many other types of similar incidents. All of these acts may cause subluxation or stresses on their bodies.

If left untreated, the subluxation may lead to a variety of common injuries, ailments and disorders including:

- Ear Aches and Ear Infections
- ADD / ADHD
- Bed Wetting
- Asthma
- Tonsillitis
- Stomach Aches
- Autism
- Allergies

You will find many stories in this book from parents whose toddlers were suffering from the conditions listed above. Once we examined the toddlers and discovered the underlying cause of their problems, we were able to remove the subluxation with our gentle and safe chiropractic adjustments.

Toddlers are some of our best patients! They are fast learners and seem to be in better touch with their bodies than at any other stage of life. In fact, we have many parents tell us when their toddlers feel something isn't quite right with their bodies; they tell their mom or dad that it's time to go see Dr. Baker.

6
Chiropractic Care for Pre-Teens and Teens

Junior high and high school students are under a lot of pressure including stress, dramatic growth and hormonal changes. This is a stage of life and a generation that thrives on technology.

Puberty is known for awkwardness, self consciousness and coordination issues. These are also the years associated with intense sports activities for both boys and girls subjecting them to all types of situations that may lead to subluxation and injuries.

Many teens suffer back pain and posture problems from carrying around backpacks filled with heavy books and their intense use of technological devices like smart phones, tablets and laptops.

We have seen with our teenage patients how regular chiropractic care benefits them and helps them deal with the radical physical, emotional and hormonal changes they are experiencing.

Our chiropractic care provides solutions for common conditions found in the teenage years including:

- Sports injuries
- Scoliosis
- Acne
- Headaches
- Cramping
- Eating Disorders
- Joint Pain
- Muscle Pain
- Back Pain
- Poor Posture and Forward Head Posture along with Text Neck

In today's world of technology and texting, Text Neck is a term that has been coined to describe the headaches, neck pain, shoulder pain and back pain that manifests from poor posture and the stress on the body created by frequently using mobile devices.

However, the condition has been around since way before the first cell phone. Text Neck is the modern day term for the more classical health condition known as Forward Head Posture.

It's important for all teens to understand the importance of good posture and a healthy spine. The health and wellness of their future depends on it.

7
Chiropractic Care
for Young Adults

Adulthood brings with it a very busy lifestyles filled with things like continuing education, a career, relationships, starting a family as well as many, many long hours.

Because of hectic schedules and demands, young adults often give other things priority instead of taking care of themselves.

These are very important years to provide your body with sufficient exercise, proper nutrition and the many benefits of a healthy spine and nervous system. Taking care of your body during these crucial years and developing healthy habits will have a significant impact on your quality of life as you age.

For more than 20 years, we have been helping our young adult patients with a variety of conditions including:

19

- Stress
- Back Pain
- Carpal Tunnel Syndrome
- Neck Pain
- Joint Pain
- Muscle Pain
- Headaches
- Infertility
- Pregnancy
- Anxiety
- Depression
- Fibromyalgia
- Sciatica
- Irritable Bowel Syndrome
- Much more!

We have included numerous stories in this book from our young adult patients who were battling a variety of painful health conditions. As you read these stories, note how many of their issues started in their teenage years and went left untreated. Just think how they could have avoided those problems had they been introduced to chiropractic care at a very young age.

Also notice in their stories how once they got out of pain and became educated they began to change their lifestyles and started incorporating the 5 Essentials of the Baker Chiropractic and Wellness Maximized Lifestyle into their daily lives.

8
Chiropractic Care
for Active Adults

Active adults and Baby Boomers are not immune to ailments, injuries, disorders and disease. In fact, since Baby Boomers make up about 30% of the population in the United States, there is a good chance you may be suffering from some type of pain or health condition. That's why our chiropractic care is so important.

Most active adult Baby Boomers are retired or have reduced their work schedules and want to continue to live life to the fullest. That means an active lifestyle focused on spending more time with your children and grandchildren, traveling, socializing with friends, participating in hobbies or perhaps even starting a whole new career.

21

Whatever your plans may be, the right exercise and nutrition along with our chiropractic care are key elements to enjoying this special time in your life.

We've helped thousands of active adults with painful conditions like:

- Arthritis
- Osteoporosis
- Back Pain
- Failed Back Surgery
- Neck Pain
- Stress
- Anxiety
- Depression
- Fibromyalgia
- Muscle Pain
- Headaches
- Much, much more

Our active adult patients have submitted many real-life stories found within the pages of this book about how they got out of pain and on the road to health and wellness. It's never too late to find solutions for your painful health conditions and change your future for the better!

9
Chiropractic Care for Seniors

Our bodies will age. That's something we just can't stop. However, your senior years do not need to be a period of time dependent on prescription medications, hospitals and nursing homes.

The chiropractic care we provide is instrumental in helping seniors eliminate pain, increase flexibility, enhance strength and maintain balance.

Our guidance with proper exercise, nutrition and therapy will also aid overall health and wellness.

Live life to the very fullest, independently and on your terms. We have helped our patients live vibrant lives throughout their senior years!

10
Chiropractic Care for the Entire Family

I grew up with my mom having the occasional back problems from a car accident in her youth. She would get treatment from a chiropractor and the only results that I ever recall observing was my mom tapping the refrigerator

magnets along her spine because the chiropractor told her magnets will help heal and put "things" back in place. So, my early impression was you go to a chiropractor only for back problems and magnets was the extent of the treatment. Little did I know...

In the fall of 2016, my mom fell down the stairs and she unknowingly injured her shoulder and neck when she held onto the banister to catch herself. Within a few months of her fall, she could barely lift her arm. Her doctor referred her to see a chiropractor. My mom did her research and she found the *"Best of the Best"* chiropractor in Cincinnati to make sure she got the best possible care. The chiropractor she found was Baker Chiropractic and Wellness on Red Bank Road.

Over the Christmas Holiday, the whole family got together to talk about how we all are and what is new, etc. During this conversation, I was giving my sister-in-law a neck and shoulder massage to work out several huge tension knots that were causing her severe pain and discomfort. Of course my mom, being the wonderful nurturer that she is, wanted to help. She shared her story with us and the progress she made at Baker Chiropractic and Wellness.

Mom told my sister-in-law that Baker Chiropractic was having this amazing holiday special. $21 to get your assessment, x-rays and your first adjustment and encouraged my sister-in-law to make an appointment for the next morning.

My sister-in-law has always had back issues. She broke her back playing competitive soccer in high school and has had sciatic issues ever since. My brother threw his back out about six months prior and still had some residual pain. So, my sister-in-law and brother went to Baker Chiropractic and Wellness the next morning, both taking advantage of the special, and came back with glowing reviews.

My sister-in-law told us how our neck is supposed to be at a 43 degree curve and that her neck was in the negatives. I immediately thought, well if her number is that bad, I know I had to be much worse, since I have horrible posture and the start of a bump on my back. My sister-in-law then showed us this diagram that lists all the things the spine affects. We start going thru the list and all our minds were blown. It was like going thru a checklist of all our aches, pains and random ailments. Therefore, with a combination of my mom, my sister-in-law and my brother saying it was worth it, my sister and I made our appointments.

I have had back pain since my junior year of high school. I was at swim practice one day and suddenly I had shooting pain up and down my spine. I went to the emergency room to see what was wrong. They did several tests and x-rays but they couldn't find anything wrong. I was told since there is nothing wrong, go home, take some ibuprofen and put some ice on it. My back was never the same. I would go through periods of it being fine and just be a dull ache, but then I would bend down, lean too far, pick-up something too heavy, sleep weird, whatever and Bing, there is the shooting pain again. I never would know what would trigger it. I would avoid anything I thought would cause it flair up especially when the ache escalated to a twinge. I knew it was agitated then and I had I to be careful.

Some of my other ailments was that I had been experiencing mysterious nerve issues in my hands. I would have random numbness in my pinky and ring fingers. They would also lock up for no apparent reason. I also suffered from self-diagnosed restless leg syndrome in my left leg. I even had unexplained tummy issues. When I would eat something, sometimes it would be fine, and then sometimes it wouldn't. I had also lost my sense of smell.

January 4, 2017 was my first appointment. It fit in quite nicely with my new year's resolution to actually start going to see doctors and get healthy. My appointment was with Dr. Todd Worthington and he was great. He really explained everything to me in detail. He not only answered all of my questions, but he answered them in layman's terms.

I was shocked to find out how messed up my back truly was. I had subluxations in 5 areas of my spine, hitting 4 of the 5 plexus and the cranial nerves. Basically, my entire nervous system was being affected. My neck was at -3 degrees instead of the 43 degrees, my lower back was over curved, my hips were uneven causing scoliosis in several places, making my spine look like it zig zags, plus disc deterioration in multiple places.

So needless to say, I was a hot mess and I had no clue. I was a little overwhelmed but Dr. Todd was very encouraging saying all of this was reversible, it wasn't some kind of final sentencing. He said with a lot of hard work and commitment, we can turn things around.

We hit the ground running with my treatment plan, I went 3 times week for 3 months. With the combination of the therapy, adjustments and the home kit, I got better. The body is a wonderful thing, it autocorrects as much as possible. But that can be a bad thing too because it is hard to tell when things are wrong. I had no idea I was so off, because feeling off was the norm for me. But once I started to get aligned and my body was being put back together correctly, I felt amazing. I have never felt so healthy and strong. I would call my normal everyday feeling was blah and sickly and I had no idea that is how I was really feeling. I thought it was fine and good. But now thanks to Dr. Todd and Baker Chiropractic I know better. I know what it feels like to really feel good.

My numbers have improved, I am now at 5 degrees on my neck,

my hips have leveled out so I am not so zig zaggy, and my posture has improved, I haven't had a back flare up since my treatment started, I am down to the very dull ache and the occasional twinge if I push myself to far. I didn't get sick like I do every winter, my sense of smell has improved and I just feel healthy, like the way my body was designed to feel.

My treatment isn't finished; I still have a long way to go before I am 100%. I have had my own challenges with bump on my back and that will take time to reverse. This is in conjunction with getting my neck to 43 degrees. It has been hindered due to in my second month of treatment, I had my own tumble down a set of stairs and injured my shoulder and neck too. But I was fortunate that I had an appointment the next morning to immediately start work on my shoulder and neck. If I hadn't been going to a chiropractor, I would have ended up similar to my mom and not being able to lift my arm. So, I did a few steps back, but I never lost the momentum forward and I will continue to do so.

This has been a whole family affair for us and we are so grateful to everyone at Baker Chiropractic and Wellness who have help all of us on our journey. We are a healthier and happier family because of their knowledgeable expertise. I would recommend them to everyone.

You never know how much better things could be unless you try!

— **Katrina A.**

· · · · ·

Where to begin? Dr. Patrick, chiropractic care and the Maximized Life style have impacted our family in so many ways. It all began about a year and a half ago in February of 2013. My husband's boss was being treated by Baker Chiropractic and seeing improvements in many areas of his life. He was so convinced of the benefits of chiropractic care that he suggested we give it a try as well. He told us of many patients he heard talking about how much it had helped their children with ADD/ADHD as well as kids who were patients so excited about their own improvements. Our teenage son, Jake, has ADHD and had been on medication since he was in 2nd grade for this as well as seasonal allergies. So we decided that we would at least check into it for ourselves as well as for our son.

As you will hear many people say...we were very skeptical. My husband, Gary, was having some back, neck and shoulder pain and bouts with acid reflux that he was treating more and more frequently with medication. He also developed a pretty annoying case of vertigo. I have had several knee surgeries and as a result have felt "out of balance" which caused some lower back, hip and even neck pain. I also have tennis elbow that bothers me from time to time and had been struggling with it for over a year and just couldn't get relief. So again, with much skepticism, we decided to give Baker Chiropractic a try.

Right off the bat we were impressed with how well they explained everything to you. They talked about how chiropractic care works, what causes problems, why doing what they do helps and what your treatment plan would be. They do x-rays and other tests that show you concrete proof of what is wrong with your spine and how they plan to correct it. We could see how chiropractic care could help with aches and pains but through educating their patients we began to understand how it could also help so many other things such as ADHD, acid reflux, headaches, allergies, vertigo, etc.

By April of 2013 we stopped giving Jake his ADHD medication as well as his seasonal allergy medication. A few times over the previous 9 years we had tried to stop the ADHD medication with no success. I am happy to say that he has now been off ALL medication for 15 months! He is a much happier kid and we are much happier parents. Having to give your child medication everyday was never what we wanted. I wish we would have known what a difference seeing a chiropractor would have made for him so much sooner. He is now 17 and is so convinced of the benefits of chiropractic care and loves it so much that he told Dr. Patrick he wanted to work for him someday. To his surprise Doc asked him to join the team this spring and Jake has found a new path for his life. We are now looking into undergraduate school and then Palmer College of Chiropractic in four years. I think he has found his passion and what he wants to do with the rest of his life. I can't even explain the positive impact Dr. Patrick has had on Jake! He is a great doctor but also a very kind and caring person. All of the staff is. Jake primarily works with Dr. Brock and he has taken him under his wing and has been instrumental in not only Jake's health but also his passion for his work. The love for what they do is clear every time you are there. I have never seen either of the docs in a bad mood. The atmosphere is always cheerful and happy. I think surrounding yourself with this kind of energy adds another level to healing and health.

Gary and I have also seen much success with Dr. Patrick. Gary has almost no lower back, shoulder or neck pain. He has not taken any acid reflux medication since we have been receiving treatment. And the vertigo is almost completely gone. My tennis elbow was gone after just a few visits and my aches and pains have almost all disappeared. I say almost because we all sleep funny or twist something occasionally and have some pains but a few adjustments later and you are feeling like a million bucks. Another pleasant surprise was relief from migraines. I was not one to have migraines all the time but I did get them once a month to a few times a month. I have had a total of 2 in the last year and a half!

After seeing the improvements the three of us were realizing we talked our oldest daughter, Becca, into giving it a try as well. She had been suffering from severe headaches for quite some time. She had trips to the emergency room, visits to the family doctor, neurologists, and a multitude of tests and medications that gave her no relief or good explanation as to the cause of her headaches. She was away at college at the time so coming in for frequent visits was kind of difficult but she visited the Doc when she was home on break or home for a short visits and of course while she was home for the summer. She saw improvements in her headaches right away. She is still away at school and was not home over the summer so hasn't been able to squeeze in as many visits as she would like but she still sees much improvement in the frequency and severity of her headaches. I am convinced if she were able to receive adjustments on a more regular basis she would be completely headache free. She is still quite happy with the improvement thus far.

This brings us to the final member of our family, Libbi. She has been a competitive volleyball player since she was 9 years old. She is now entering her sophomore year playing for Thomas More College. She is very active and has stayed pretty fit but the wear and tear of her workouts for so many years had lead to some back pain. She was the last one to jump on the chiropractic care band wagon as quite honestly she thought it looked a little scary. She was nervous but finally decide to give it a try when her back was really bothering her and limiting some of her work outs. With her schedule, being away at college and volleyball she was also limited in the number of visits she could squeeze in. She saw immediate improvements and now squeezes adjustments in whenever she is home for visits as well as regular appointments over the summer. Her last X-rays show an almost picture perfect spine and she is very proud of that and feeling great!!

And now for the last way Baker Chiropractic has impacted our lives. Gary and I have talked about trying to change the way we eat for years. We both felt like eating healthier would make us feel better as well as help us lose weight. Our attempts at weight loss or eating healthy through the years were not very successful. Trying to navigate the grocery store and food packaging to try to figure what was healthy or good to eat was overwhelming. When Jake started working for Baker in the spring he also decided he wanted to try to eat healthier. Doc sent him home with the book he and his brother wrote: What Did I Just Eat. I started to read the book and couldn't put it down. I finished it the next morning and that afternoon cleaned out our pantry and refrigerator. We have been eating a much healthier whole food diet. We have cut out sugar, refined salt and processed food, among other things. At first you think that sounds impossible to do but it really isn't that hard. You see improvements in how you feel very quickly and weight loss happens as a pleasant side effect so continuing to eat healthy is pretty easy. We still have days that are not so healthy....vacation, family get togethers, etc.

While these breaks are kind of fun occasionally, you see that you don't feel as well afterwards so getting back on track to healthy eating is not a problem. We feel better over all and Gary has lost 20 lbs. I have lost 30 lbs so far.

As you can see....Dr. Patrick, Dr. Brock and the Baker staff have had a very large impact on the quality of life in the Giuliano family. We are all very thankful for the wonderful care we have received and the improvements we feel daily. We are very happy to be part of the Baker family!

— **Patti G.**

• • • • •

11
Acid Reflux (GERD)

I decided to get chiropractic work done because I am on my third pregnancy and had a lot of back pain and hip pain. It was incredibly uncomfortable and my acid reflux was awful.

I've only been here now about 4 visits, and I am feeling absolutely no back pain or hip pain! My acid reflux has diminished quite a bit too and now pains that I didn't even realize were there are diminishing as well!

I'm feeling a lot better, my sleep is no longer disrupted, and my mood towards my family is better. I can move around better, and I am not "waddling" as much. I am walking more.

Thank you Dr. Mike and Baker Chiropractic!

— Mandy T.

• • • • •

"I started coming to Baker Chiropractic because I was having a lot of indigestion and pain in my middle back. In 2 months time, my indigestion is gone and I no longer have middle back pain."

— **Justine**

• • • • •

"A few months ago my infant daughter, was having severe gas pains regularly and she wasn't pooping very often. I took her into the Pediatrician when she was 4 months old and he said that it was normal for some breastfed babies to go 7-10 days between bowel movements and that she was okay. Then, when she was 5 months old, I took her to another Pediatrician since the problem had not gone away and was worse. I wanted to know what I could do to alleviate her pain. The doctor said that I should start her on regular foods (which I had put off starting because of the problem) and that the problem would most likely correct itself within the next month! So, there I was with a five-month-old child who was having horrible gas pains on a daily basis and she wanted me to wait a whole month for things to get better! I was really upset because this had already been going on for quite some time and we were at a point when neither of us could take it anymore. She was in pain and so was I because I hated to hear my baby cry when I couldn't do anything to help her.

So, I asked my chiropractor, Dr. Paul Baker, if he thought he might be able to help me. He said he'd be more than happy to adjust her and he was confident he could help, so I brought her in. I was very hopeful, but didn't really know what to expect. Dr. Paul adjusted her back and neck and that night she pooped! We were thrilled because it had been so long since she had done that. I brought her in one week later and again, she pooped that night. Then she pooped the next morning and a couple more times that week. I went back each week for about 6 weeks and things just kept getting better and better. It really only took four adjustments before she was perfectly normal again. She is now a pooping machine and I couldn't be happier. She is 9 months old and as happy as can be! I can't remember the last time she had gas pains! It's a wonderful thing! I very much appreciate Dr. Paul and how great he is with my whole family and I'm grateful he was there to help me at a time when the Pediatricians didn't know what to do. It was truly an answer to our prayers."

— **Rachel**

. . . . .

It has been about three years; I can actually say that I enjoy my weekly visits to Dr. Baker's office. Not only has he kept me pretty well pain free, but there has been an added perk with help with my acid reflux issue. I cannot tell you in this short testimonial how many things these doctors can help people with, all without the need for medications and/or surgeries.

Kudos again to you and your staff, Dr. Baker!

— **J. Smith**

. . . . .

12
ADD / ADHD and Anti-Depressants

I first found Baker Chiropractic after injuring my back. I was standing on a patch of ice while lifting my 5 year old into her car seat. I started to slide and twisted in an odd direction to avoid dropping my daughter. I felt an odd sensation in my back when I fell then the pain started. I spent two days in bed using ice and heating pads. Nothing was helping. I had always been rather skeptical chiropractics believing it was gimmicky nonsense. At this point though with 3 young children and being in such pain I became desperate. I made my appointment and met with Dr. Baker still quite skeptical. When my adjustment was over I was amazed at the relief I felt. I was able to move again. I admit I was shocked how well it worked.

My mother suffered from a lot of neck, back and joint pain. After hearing and seeing how much I was helped by my adjustment she decided to give it a try as well. Very skeptical at first she has now become a regular at Baker Chiropractics.

After being a client for a while Dr Baker told me about how chiropractic care can help ADD & ADHD. Unwilling to medicate my 5 year old for her ADD, I decided to start bringing her in for adjustments as well. She loves Dr. Baker and her adjustments. She talks about how they make her feel better.

My 88 year old grandmother lives overseas in the Netherlands. She suffers from major neck pain due to degeneration. Dr Baker has started giving her adjustments when she visits us. After trying everything in The Netherlands from injections in the neck to deaden the nerves to major pain killers we have finally found something that helps her pain, adjustments at Baker Chiropractic.

Now nearly a year later Dr Baker is now treating 4 generations of women in my family. I am very happy I found Baker Chiropractic.

— M. Murphy

· · · · ·

There I was last summer, coping with months of unemployment and no prospects for work. My adolescent son found refuge from the stress and uncertainty through video gaming. When he wasn't gaming, he was oppositional and agitated. He lived on soda and snacks, lost interest in sports, friends and swimming at the neighborhood pool. His posture deteriorated after spending weeks of summer vacation hunched over the laptop on the floor, addicted to an internet game.

I was busy working up resumes and cover letters, trying to score a job interview. I became concerned at how withdrawn and miserable my son was. He complained of low back and neck pain and not being able to sleep. He didn't want to attend 7th grade and exhibited mounting social and behavioral problems. He was skipping gym class, being bullied by classmates and his back pain grew increasingly worse. I did not want to have more drugs added to the ADHD medications and Anti- Depressants my son was already prescribed.

Years earlier, I had experienced positive results from chiropractic care. I wasn't sure if adolescents could benefit, but began searching for a doctor of chiropractic. I made an appointment with Dr. Paul Baker to have my son's back checked.

Dr. Baker and the staff at Baker Chiropractic transformed my son!

In less than a year, he has become positive, involved with his friends and has developed a self esteem that hasn't existed before. He no longer has continuous back and neck pain; he sleeps well and looks forward to his weekly chiropractic adjustments.

Our life has been positively infused in so many ways through the comprehensive care we both receive at Baker Chiropractic.

We now focus on wellness; from what we put into our body nutritionally, to eliminating the defeatist mindset that had invaded everyday living. Our goal is to no longer use the pharmaceuticals we had relied on to manage the symptoms caused by subluxations in our spine.

I am now happily employed and my son is a successful 8th

grader. Our health and well being have become an integral to a happy life and our future is so much brighter.

Our lifestyle transformation is the direct result of chiropractic care from Dr. Paul Baker and his encouraging and caring staff. If you are receptive to the power of positivity and the healing that result from a subluxation free spine, Baker Chiropractic can change your life.

— K. Flick

· · · · ·

When I first came to see Dr. Baker I was lazy and got bad grades in school. I was getting into trouble all the time and not listening to my teachers. My report card was real bad and my parents were very frustrated with me. I was taking tons of medications for my ADD and ADHD. First I was on Ritalin. Then I took Concerta. I was also on Medadate and Zoloft.

Since I began treatment with Dr. Baker, I've been able to get off all my medications and actually feel like a human being again.

I used to walk around feeling like I was stoned and in another world. I was depressed and flunking school. Now, I feel super and on top of the world.

I can't thank Dr. Baker enough for all his help in changing my life.

— K. Mason

· · · · ·

I found out about Baker Chiropractic from another parent on my sons football team. The parent approached me and politely pointed out that he noticed my son ran awkwardly and was one of the slowest kids on the team. When Kasey was two he fell and broke his femur. He was put in a body cast for two months. After the cast

came off he had to learn how to sit up, crawl and walk again. I noticed right away that something wasn't right about the way he moved and that he did not like to run. We went to different medical doctors about it several times. The answer was always the same, "He will outgrow it."

Also around the same time he broke his leg he started having asthma attacks in his sleep. It was to the point I would have to run hot steamy showers to get him to stop coughing. We also thought Kasey was a hard headed child that would not listen to anything we asked him to do. Come to find out he had so much fluid build up behind his ear drums that he could not hear us. They put tubes in his ears to drain the fluid but he continued to have ear infections at least once a month. Kasey also struggled with school work. He knew the answers to questions but was not able to process them from his mind to paper. He had a hard time blending sounds when reading simple stories.

We decided to take this parents advice to go see Dr. Baker. Come to find out Kasey's upper spine was out which was connected to his ears and his thinking process. His lower spine was also out from breaking his leg. Kasey has been seeing Dr. Baker for 2 years now and it is amazing the difference we see in him. He now loves to run hasn't had an asthma attack or an ear infection in 2 years and has brought his grades up in school from needing assistance in every subject to now being above average on most subjects. Kasey is now reading chapter books. Has a 100% in Math. He loves to play football, basketball and baseball. We are so proud of him.

Before we started taking him to see Dr. Baker, Kasey's self esteem was extremely low after everything he had been through. Now he is extremely happy, loves all sports and full of energy. We are very thankful for Dr. Baker and everything he has done for Kasey. I would and have recommended Dr. Baker to several friends. Thank you Dr. Baker.

— **The Cook Family**

13
Allergies

I met Dr. Patrick Baker through BEAT Personal Training. My family wanted to help me lose and control my weight gain and recommended me to BEAT.

My younger sister actually made my first appointment for me and forced me to go. I talked to Dr. Patrick Baker one day after my workout

because I was experiencing pain and numbness in my legs when I did certain exercises or sat on the floor. I also told him about my ATV accident from 6 years ago. Dr. Baker told me he could help me, said to come see him in his office and he would take care of it. So I did. That was almost two years ago.

Dr. Baker is slowly straightening my "s" shaped spine and I am reaping the benefits of chiropractic care.

I like to boast about the lack of allergies and sinus problems the most. I was prone to sinus infections 2-3 times a year and had severe allergies throughout the change of seasons. I am very happy to tell everyone I meet that chiropractic care helped reduce my allergies and sinus problems.

I am a very satisfied patient and have referred several people, including my father, sister, and brother-in-law (all patients now).

My heartfelt thanks goes out to Dr. Baker and staff.

— **Michelle T.**

• • • • •

Early one morning, I sent a message to Baker Chiropractic and Wellness. By 4:00 pm that same afternoon I started on my road to recovery.

Over 10 years ago, I began having chronic ear and sinus infections. I have 2 older sisters and they both began having ear infections around the same age. They both had PE tubes placed and never had issues with ear infections again.

My primary care doctor treated the infections for a while and then recommended that I see an Ear, Nose & Throat specialist. The first ENT told me that adults don't get chronic ear infections. Basically, he totally blew me off. No treatment was provided!

I found another ENT and was taken seriously. Unfortunately, his interventions did not lead to success. He recommended PE tubes and they worked for about 6 months. Even with the tubes, I had 2 additional ear infections. The last ear infection resulted in the tubes being displaced. The ENT allowed my ears to "heal" and started me on an allergy medication. He also recommended that I see an allergist. I began a long road of twice a week allergy injections. The only thing that I received from the allergy injections was that I no longer have a fear of needles!

Next, the ENT recommended sinus surgery for new, more permanent PE tube placement, and to repair to my deviated septum. I would not recommend sinus surgery to anyone! It was extremely painful and took almost a month to recover from.

About a month after surgery, the ENT figured out why I was taking so long to recovery! I developed Methicillin-resistant Staphylococcus aureus (MRSA). My follow up CAT scan showed that the sinus surgery was not successful. Due to the infection, more scar tissue had formed in my nose and sinuses. His recommendation? Let's do the surgery again! I told him that I needed time to consider my options.

About 2 months later, I woke up in excruciating pain. I called my ENT and was informed that he was no longer in practice. I called my PCP and she was able to find me another ENT. The PE tubes, placed two months prior, were no longer in the place. He removed the tubes from the ear canal and told me to see him in 3 months.

My PCP finally decided that I should see a SINUS guy! I was thrilled that I would finally get relief from chronic pain and pressure. I had another CAT scan done. All my hopes were short lived. The ENT looked at my CAT scan and said that "if I was looking for surgery then I came to the wrong doctor." Surgery was the last thing on my mind. But to get relief, I would have gladly had another surgery! The doctor then recommended that I take allegra and a saline spray daily. He assured me that this would relieve all my symptoms!

A year later, he was dead wrong! In this past year alone, I have seen a doctor over 20 times! All visits were for my ears or sinuses. Even after all those visits, I still had chronic sinus pain and pressure. That pressure led to multiple ear infections in the past year.

After too many sleepless nights, I searched and found Baker Chiropractic and Wellness and submitted an appointment request at 4:00 am. I received a response from Danielle by 8:00 am with an appointment that same day. I was impressed from the moment I walked in the door. Everyone was friendly and professional. I got my first adjustment and was amazed that I had some relief. A month later, I have no ear pain! Sinuses are a work in progress but I have 100% faith that they will get better!

My x-rays showed some low back degeneration. I am a nurse and have assumed that back pain was part of the job! I am thrilled to say it is no longer part of the job! Dr. Patrick Baker is heaven sent! He provided me with a thorough understanding of the purpose of chiropractic care and what my x-rays showed. His warm, caring approach is wonderful! I cannot say enough good things about Dr. Baker and the staff at the West Chester, Ohio Chiropractic Clinic!

Their caring and compassion go beyond anything I have ever experienced! I recently experienced a death of a loved one and was overwhelmed by the support I received from Baker Chiropractic. From a thoughtful touch to a sympathy card, Baker Chiropractic went above and beyond to share my loss. I have never had a doctor that knows so much about me and truly cares!

— **Valerie H.**

• • • • •

I started seeing Dr. Brock Frear at Baker Chiropractic and Wellness in June of 2014 after developing severe pain in my lower back and sciatic nerve.

I was about 3 weeks away from a trip to Hawaii and did not want to waste time with traditional medicine which would involve medications and worse yet possible surgery.

Within several weeks my back was doing great and eventually felt better than ever. I had read many articles and talked with Dr. Brock about how chiropractic care enables the body to heal itself of many ailments.

I didn't think too much of that until the spring of 2015 when I realized, unlike the past several years, I did not suffer from spring seasonal allergies that seemed to be worsening each year. This was one of the worst allergy seasons and I work outside all day.

I am a firm believer that my regular adjustments prevented me from suffering the effects of allergies this spring.

This time last year I never would have believed chiropractic care could do that but today there is no doubt this works.

— Jeff D

• • • • •

I started coming to Baker Chiropractic and Wellness a little more than two years ago. I was experiencing pain with head movement of any kind. I had also been having periods of vertigo over the previous few years. After speaking with my regular doctor about the neck pain and if there was a connection between it and the vertigo, I was not satisfied with her solution of taking medications. That is when I decided to give

chiropractic care a try. I was nervous about having someone work with my neck, but something needed to be done about the pain.

Treatment started with an exam and X-ray. I was actually listened to as I explained what was happening with my neck. It was so refreshing to talk with someone who cared and understood. The

X-rays showed the curve in my neck was basically non-existent. He promised that chiropractic treatments could help me. Over the past two years, it really has.

The chiropractic adjustments and treatments started bringing relief to my pain right away. These were combined with recommended home exercises which I still do twice a day. Each follow-up X-ray showed improvement in the curvature of my neck. I was experiencing more neck motion with less pain.

Since starting chiropractic care, there have been no new episodes of vertigo. If I am feeling any change in ear pressure, I let them know at adjustment time. It really helps. I used to experience an average of three headaches a month. Since starting treatment, I have only had a few headaches in the last two years.

An unexpected benefit of chiropractic care has been a huge improvement in my allergies. After moving to Ohio 30 years ago, I started having really bad allergies every spring and fall. It was so bad that I had to use a prescription antihistamine like Zyrtek and Flonase nasal spray. Often I would develop a sinus or ear infection as well. The medications were able to stop the allergy symptoms, but they left me feeling tired all the time. I have not had to take a single antihistamine or use nasal spray in the last two years! I would not say my allergies have completely disappeared, but they have decreased to the point where I can actually live without medication except an occasional decongestant. I have not had any sinus or ear infections either. I no longer have to dread months of feeling like I am living in a medicine fog.

The quality of my life has improved so much since coming to Baker Chiropractic. No matter how I am feeling each time I go, I always leave feeling better. I encourage anyone who is suffering to give them a try. I highly recommend them!

— Jean W

· · · · ·

14
Arthritis

My name is Marlene and I was at the point of thinking "If this is what growing old is like, it's no fun!"

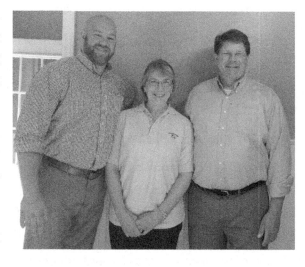

I had neck pain and back problems for 20+ years. I always felt sick and was unable to look up or turn my head. I couldn't do things I enjoy like gardening or slow dancing. I couldn't hug anyone or turn my head to chat with someone.

I started chiropractic care as a last chance before having to undergo neck surgery. When I started to see signs of recovery with chiropractic care, I knew this was the answer and I wanted total and complete recovery.

Not only did I get mobility back with my neck and back but I found I could now lay on my right side without immediate dizziness.

Recently, my family doctor said I had arthritis in my wrists. Oh my aching hands. Dr. Joe Fields took a look and fixed them with just one adjustment. He takes care of my wrists every week now. No more aching!

After chiropractic care at Baker Chiropractic and Wellness, I can now:

- Look up
- Hug people
- Lay down however I want without dizziness
- Turn my head from side-to-side
- Hold my head up

I also had no idea chiropractic care could fix my aching hands and in the last two weeks, I can breath with my mouth closed. No more snoring!

I got my life back. I can live because I can move!

My name is Tim and I had been struggling with headaches, lower back pain and hip problems for a few years. I was diagnosed with osteoarthritis and given pain killers for the hip pain. I eventually had both hips replaced and I couldn't do much of anything.

The chiropractic care I have received at Baker Chiropractic and Wellness gives me energy, mobility and just makes me feel better overall. I would not be able to work 12+ hour days without chiropractic care. I am also sick far less and haven't had a case of the flu since coming here.

— Marlene and Tim M.

• • • • •

After a knee replacement last summer I thought I was finally going to resume my busy life pain free. Over the last ten years arthritis had made its claim on me and resulted in two back surgeries, two foot surgeries, an ankle surgery and two knee surgeries. After years of suffering I made the decision to have a knee replacement and thought it was going to be the answer to my physical challenges. I wanted to reclaim my active lifestyle as a teacher, performer and sports enthusiast. The knee replacement itself was successful, but approximately two months after recovering from the surgery I began having horrific back and leg pain again. This time I was determined to find an answer without surgery. My son, who is studying to be a chiropractor himself, insisted that I go to a chiropractor.

So, with some hesitation and uncertainty, in January of 2011 I sought treatment with Dr. Baker. I remember my first several visits being overcome with emotion. Dr. Baker and his staff were warm and welcoming; I immediately felt they genuinely cared. They gave me hope. I was impressed with the patient education and realized how uninformed I was regarding the whole realm of chiropractic care. It was clear that treatment would take time and would require patience and a commitment on my part. After the first few treatments I could feel a difference. I improved more and more with each visit. Now, after eight months, I feel stronger and healthier than I have in years and plan to continue chiropractic care as a way of life.

So how has chiropractic care changed my life? I'm back on the golf course, riding my bike, and enjoying roller coasters again. I'm able to walk long distances and run up stairs. I'm performing on stage without pain for the first time in years. But it is in my profession as a music teacher where I have felt the most dramatic results of my treatment. I'll never forget the afternoon one of my sweet second grade boys smiled at me after we had just been dance partners in class. The innocent sincerity of his words warmed my heart and will remain etched in my memory. "I am so happy you can dance with us again, Mrs. Lewis." Thank you, Dr. Baker. Thank you for giving me my life back!

— **M. Lewis**

• • • • •

15
Asthma

I have been living here in Ohio for the past 3 years and I have seen 8 different chiropractors.

I am a hard person to adjust because I have been in a few accidents that left me, on two separate occasions, unable to walk.

Not one chiropractor here has been able to "get all of me in", until I found Dr. Baker.

Dr. Baker was able to adjust my neck, middle and lower back unlike the other 8 different chiropractors!

What a great feeling! For the first time in 3 long years I could feel the difference in my body. I cannot describe how good that feeling is.

I never have a headache, my asthma is under control now, I

stand up straighter and even my vision has improved.

Before chiropractic, I thought I had to live in chronic pain, now I have seen the difference in myself.

My quality of life has improved and I am grateful for it.

Sincerely,
— **Debbie P.**

· · · · ·

My daughter's name is Isabella Sanchez. She was born in August 2011. When she was three months old she became very sick with asthma. We were in the ER constantly because she couldn't breathe. The Doctors put her on steroids and inhalers and antibiotics. She was constantly sick.

After 6 months of what seemed like a hopeless and exhausting situation- my friend Angela told me that I should take her to Dr. Paul Baker, with Baker Chiropractic. When she was first examined by Dr. Paul, he told me that he has never seen a baby with so many subluxations (Subluxations are the misalignment of the spine). He told me that these subluxations were the cause of her asthma and other problems.

After a few adjustments, I could tell the difference rather quickly. She wasn't as sick and in need of as much oxygen at night. After 3 months of adjustments, she was a different girl. She was asthma free and walking. She wasn't anywhere close to walking when we started with Dr. Paul. We continue to bring her in for her weekly adjustments. We are grateful to Dr. Paul Baker for helping our little girl. She is now a happy little 18 month old toddler. We owe that to Dr. Paul!

— **Isabella's Dad**

· · · · ·

My lower back really started bothering me in February of this year (I thought I pulled something when I moved into my new house.)WRONG!

My family doctor gave me muscle relaxers, pain pills, and anti inflammatory. After a week or two with no relief, he changed the medications around and I was still receiving no relief. I was in complete agony for almost three months. A co-worker told me about Dr. Baker. I called that day, May 3, 2010 and got in that same day. After reviewing my x-rays, I found out I had many problems (not from my move) subluxation, degeneration, and pinched nerves in my lumbar. Along with all of that my hips were off!

I have to admit, the first three weeks of coming here were very difficult. I really did not know if I could continue but what kept me going were the stories that I was hearing from other patients while I was waiting to get adjusted. It is amazing how many people Doc has done wonders for.

57

After three weeks of coming three times a week I started having a little relief. Here it is four months later and I am so glad that I did not give up on Doc. I feel so much better, sure I have some days with a little discomfort but when that happens I just add an extra day that week to get adjusted. (I am now down to once a week!)

A couple of weeks ago I had an asthma attack. I was skeptical on where to go. It was either my asthma specialist (which was closing in 45 minutes) or go to Dr. Baker's. Danielle said, "Come here, come here!" So off to Dr. Baker's office I went. I had already used an emergency inhaler and it did not work and I started to panic which is not a good thing with asthma! While at Doc's I received EMS, roller bed, and then a massage. Massage for asthma? I said. I trusted Doc with his recommendations and after my massage with Chris and then an adjustment with Doc my lungs were totally opened! I really was amazed but I should have known he could help me, after all that's why Doc wanted to grow up and be Chiropractor. He had asthma as a child.

You will not find any other Doctor office like this one. Everyone truly is there to help everyone. They are caring, friendly, and just all around great people. Thanks to Dr. Baker, Jennifer, Danielle, Krista, Courtney, and Chris.

— S. Mazuk

· · · · ·

16
Auto Accident Injuries

I started care here at Baker Chiropractic and Wellness less than three months ago.

I was living with low back pain for five years and severe neck pain from a car accident.

It was painful to ride my horse and pick-up my grandchildren.

To deal with the pain, I used Motrin and anti-inflammatory medications.

I was skeptical about chiropractic care at first. I didn't really believe in it. I thought it was just popping and moving bones.

After the care I have received at Baker Chiropractic and

Wellness, I was able to take a 4-hour flight with absolutely no pain. I can also now ride my horse again for hours with no problem.

If I would not have come here, I would still be in pain.

I recommend that anyone who has back pain or neck pain like I did to come here and get evaluated.

— Colleen A.

• • • • •

I have been living here in Ohio the past 3 years and I have seen 8 different chiropractors. I am a hard person to adjust because I have been in a few accidents that left me on 2 separate occasions unable to walk.

Not one chiropractor here has been able to "get all of me in", until I found Dr. Baker.

Dr. Baker was able to adjust my neck, middle and lower back unlike the other 8 different chiropractors!

What a great feeling! For the first time in 3 long years I could feel the difference in my body. I cannot describe how good that feeling is.

I never have a headache, my asthma is under control now, I stand up straighter and even my vision has improved.

Before chiropractic, I thought I had to live in chronic pain, now I have seen the difference in myself.

My quality of life has improved and I am grateful for it.

Sincerely,

— **Debbie P.**

· · · · ·

My name is JoAnn and my trouble began after a car accident while I was in high school. So my issues are from long term injuries.

As time went on, years of standing at my job took a toll on my neck and back. In the early 90's, I did go see Dr. Baker and got treated with success but I stopped going.

In 2004, I went for a MRI for my neck and the specialist told me surgery was not an option. By 2009, the pain had increased to the point where I was wearing a neck brace while sleeping to get some relief.

In 2014, I went back to the specialist because the pain in my hip down down to my right foot began to burn. I felt my foot going numb. I told them about my neck injury and they said this pain was in my back and had nothing to do with my neck. I really was not comfortable with that answer. They told me to go get an MRI and see a back surgeon immediately.

I called Dr. Baker because I was hurting. I was crying in pain and his office staff could not have been more compassionate with me.

61

Dr. Baker began treating me and almost immediately the pain was relieved. He told me exactly the step by step plan I needed to follow and it is working!

This is a journey for me but what a difference! I am no longer wearing my neck brace after 2 years and my pain is going away. For the first time I can see that I am reversing what time has done to me.

Now I am standing straight, turning my neck, and have no back pain. I'm so excited I plan to join a gym and start really concentrating on getting healthy and stronger.

I thank God for sending Dr. Baker and his staff my way and showing me so much compassion when I went there in pain and tears. It's so nice to be pain free, healthy, and free from medications. This has been a real breakthrough for me!

Thanks again to Dr. Baker and the staff and the good Lord for using his team to help others.

God Bless you all,
— JoAnn S.

• • • • •

In June, I was involved in an auto accident. My back starting hurting shortly after, so I went to the hospital. The physician who was on call told me it was a "stiff back" and prescribed muscle relaxers and pain pills. Needless to say, they didn't work. They only made me sleep.

I came to Baker Chiropractic about three weeks after the accident. I was very skeptical at first because I believed chiropractic medicine was only a way for people to get rich who practiced it. Boy was I ever wrong!

In one week of treatment, the pain had diminished by 50%. I was able to do most of my regular activities. At the end of the third week, I was living life completely pain free. I really am very lucky that I became a patient of Baker Chiropractic.

— R. Hall

• • • • •

A few days after I was in an auto accident, I had excruciating pain in both my neck and head from whiplash. I was not able to turn my neck to either side; my neck and head hurt constantly. No relief was to be had. I tried numerous pain killers, but nothing helped. My mother had whiplash many years before, and only a chiropractor could help her. So I set out to find a good chiropractor. What amazing luck that I was sent by a friend to Baker Chiropractic!

From the very first adjustment, my constant headache decreased about 90%. I could now turn my neck to both sides, which previously had been impossible. Within 3 treatments, both my headaches and my neck pain stopped completely- to my great relief!

On another occasion, I had been having problems with my right shoulder. It hurt severely and I could not lift my arm over my head. No matter how much the arm hurt, I just could not move it very high. I mentioned this difficulty to Dr. Paul. Happily, he said he is a shoulder man and has helped many painful shoulders over the years. Again, I was truly lucky to have these gentlemen as my chiropractors. After the first treatment, I noticed an immense difference. My shoulder was not in constant pain any longer and I had much more mobility.

Following the Baker's program, I lost 45 pounds in a little over 2 months. Boy, do I feel better not carrying around the extra weight! I feel better than I have in years. I can move much better and more lightly.

They have given me my body back. For that, I cannot thank them enough. They truly care about each and every patient. That's a great deal to get from a health care professional.

Needless to say, they have added an immense amount to my life.

Thank you Dr. Paul and Dr. Patrick!

— S. DeRyke

. . . . .

I was in a car accident which left me with severe low back pain and hip pain. It was very hard and painful to walk or sit for long periods of time. I was also used to a routine of working out several times per week and could no longer do so. I have young children that were used to having their mother pick them up but I wasn't able to do that either. The stress of the accident and the pain caused a previous health condition of Crohn's Disease to flare.

After each adjustment at Baker Chiropractic, I was able to walk better, sit longer without pain and eventually return to exercising. I could once again pick up my children without any pain. Dr. Baker also helped slow down the progress of the Crohn's Disease.

— D. Smith

. . . . .

By Dr. Paul Baker, Dr. Patrick Baker and Hundreds of Patients

My wife and I both suffered back injuries due to accidents. She was first to discover Dr. Baker and always returned home touting his sincerity and skill. Consequently, when I became injured, it was only natural for me to seek his help.

Through the weeks and months, Baker Chiropractic has provided us with consistent care, along with a pleasant and clean atmosphere. As a result, both our physical conditions have continued to improve, and we have made great strides towards becoming pain free. Through Dr. Baker's consistent therapy, I have been able to forego pain medications for over a month now and we are ever hopeful of being able to resume the normal activities of our lives.

Dr. Baker and his caring staff went out of their way to make us feel like a part of them. Their attention to our needs has been unparalleled. Needless to say, we would recommend them in a heartbeat.

— Pastor James S. and Nichole M.

• • • • •

I had been experiencing neck pain and back pain for approximately 2-3 years. Like everyone else, I have a busy schedule and put off any treatment.

Over time, the pain would get worse as well as the lack of maneuverability. I went to a physical therapist and started receiving treatment that lasted for 10 visits. At the end of those visits, I had a series of exercises to do with the advice to continue on a daily basis until "things loosened up" then do them on an as needed basis. The problem was that a year later, I was still doing those exercises daily with little to no results. As time went on, the pain still continued to increase and simple things like getting in and out of a car became unbearable let alone not being able to keep up with my kids. So many activities became more and more limited.

I began to look for other options and researched online. This included several websites regarding chiropractic care including the chiropractor's education and experience. When I came across Baker Chiropractic Care and Wellness, I found so much information on their website, more than anyone else they answered so many questions. One of the things that caught my eye was that they centered their treatment on correcting the problem and not treating the symptoms or using medications.

Up to this point, I've never had any experience with chiropractic care and didn't think about it enough really to be skeptic. Any passing thought with this type of treatment I dismissed with little consideration. However, I called and made an appointment. When that day came, I met several employees, all of which were every bit as friendly as I read from previous testimonials.

During my initial evaluation, I was asked about headaches. I told them I get headaches frequently, not realizing this issue would be related to the condition my spine was in. Everything was explained up front as to how the treatment was customized for my situation and what I could expect.

I've been a patient at Baker Chiropractic Care and Wellness since February of 2015 and I've noticed a big difference literally after my first adjustment with Dr. Garrett Knuckles. I couldn't believe how much my maneuverability came back and how the pain decreased. What I consider a bonus is the amount of headaches I get significantly decreased as well. When I reviewed my x-rays with Dr. Garrett, it became an eye opening experience as to how serious the condition my spine was in.

After a few adjustments, I received my home care kit and exercises to do that directly relate to my condition. Unlike the exercises I received from physical therapy, these exercises actually work! The longer I've been doing them, the better the results. As I continue with my adjustments and home care, my condition is improving. I'm already able to participate with my kids in their sporting activities and perform simple tasks throughout my work day with more flexibility and less pain. I've also become more aware of sustaining a better posture with this experience and have had adjustments with Dr. Paul Baker as well.

I read the book Enlightening Adjusting and Saving Lives by Dr's. Paul and Patrick Baker. It's filled with numerous patients talking about their specific conditions and the results of their treatment. Although this book is very inspiring, I have to admit, I didn't think I would receive such results since my spine is in a phase 3 condition. However it didn't take long for me to see improvements first hand. This has inspired me to set a goal of improving my spine alignment to a phase 1 or better yet.....what would be considered a normal phase!

I don't want to think where I would be if I didn't make the call to Baker Chiropractic and Wellness. With everything I've learned so far, I would recommend everyone to give this a try and see for yourself.

Thank you Dr. Paul, Dr. Garrett, and staff!

— R. Williams

· · · · ·

I first stepped foot into Baker Chiropractic because of severe pain radiating in my neck.

I have suffered from recurring whiplash caused from bus accidents as a child that would flare up three to four times a year. I was used to experiencing the pain. But this last flare up wouldn't go away and practically debilitated me.

Three weeks later, the stabbing and throbbing pains made it difficult to work, stand, sit, and impossible to drive or sleep. Then I met the great people at Baker Chiropractic and Wellness.

Dr. Brock (Frear) took me under his wing and I saw results within a few visits. He took the time to explain his evaluation of my x¬ rays and to show me the subluxations in my spine that were the source of my pain.

In addition to the neck misalignment, Dr. Brock showed me how my hips were also out of alignment. I told him it was probably because I was babying a hurt knee. He replied that my knee was hurting because my hips were offset. He also commented on the fact that he would have thought I had issues with sciatica. My mouth dropped open as I admitted I did have on again/off again sciatic pain.

One adjustment later and I could definitely see a marked difference, not only in my neck but also in my knee. I had more range of motion in my neck, a decrease in pain, I could finally sleep at night, not to mention that I could climb stairs like a normal person again. (side note: I was not at the time suffering from sciatica so I don't know if that was solved or not – but with everything else that improved, I have no doubt that it has as well). After a couple of weeks, I felt like the old me... but better.

It's a joy to go to Baker Chiropractic and Wellness. Not only do I know that I'm correcting my health issues but also the warm and friendly atmosphere is welcoming and makes it a joy to be there. I love the holistic approach and the positivity that radiates the entire practice.

The addition of the massage therapy has helped heal the aches and pains and further preps my muscles and joints to accept the adjustments. And the home therapy gives me the tools to aid me to keep my back healthy.

Dr. Brock and all his staff have a passion for the work they are doing. They each have their own personal story to tell on how chiropractic care, specifically from Baker Chiropractic and Wellness, has enriched their lives and made their health better. It's refreshing to see people love the work they are doing....to the point where Dr. Brock says this isn't work for him and that he sees it as his joy/mission to help all of us live a happier, healthier life.

I, for one, am greatly appreciative.

I'm a true believer in Chiropractic Care from Baker Chiropractic and Wellness. I came to Baker Chiropractic to alleviate my neck pain but also found the cure for my knee and sciatic pain as well, not to mention making my other internal organs healthier. Life can't get better than that!

— **Patricia B.**

17
Back Pain

"Before going to seek treatment from Dr. Garrett Knuckles at Baker Chiropractic and Wellness, I was experiencing neck pain, lower back pain, sharp pain in my left arm and I was walking with a limp. I was also experiencing numbness in my hips which was keeping me up at night.

Dr. Garrett started me on a regiment of adjustments and in as little as four months I am now able to sleep through the night, I am practically pain free, and my limp no longer exists!

My life is so much better now thanks to Dr. Garrett and his staff!"

— **Norma S.**

· · · · ·

Dear Dr. Patrick ,

I just want to give you a great big Hallelujah shout out for your expertise. Baker Chiropractic and Wellness Center has truly been a Godsend. I originally visited your Fairfield office due to a car accident in March 2013. I was in excruciating pain and I was provided immediate relief through your specialized chiropractic care for my back, neck, and shoulder pain.

I gained such relief & energy that I was able to return to enjoying quality of life again after just a few weeks of treatment. I felt so alive after completing your recommended treatment plan in June 2013, that I decided to not return for maintenance care as you had so sincerely suggested.

Well, while on vacation In July 2016, I woke up in excruciating pain to the point that I literally could not walk or bare any weight on my lower back to left buttock and leg. The pain was radiating through my left leg to foot and I was not able to walk without assistance of someone.

As recommended by my primary physician, I was taking steroid pain medicine around the clock every 4-6 hours only to get little if any relief. Upon my return home the pain had magnified to an off the chart level. Our family physician ordered an MRI which disclosed that I had two (2) pinched nerves pressing against a bulging herniated disc. I was referred to a neurosurgeon for further evaluation regarding the results of the MRI. After a consultation meeting with a surgeon, I was advised that an epidural injection should relieve the excruciating pain; after which I would be reevaluated for possible back surgery. I had the injection on August 5, 2016, which relieved the excruciating pain but the pain returned after a few days. I still was not able to sit, stand, or walk without the assistance of someone. I was basically restricted to mostly lying down while taking pain medicine.

At the persistence of my husband, I called Baker Chiropractic and Wellness on August 9th and was advised to come into the office the next day. I entered the office with tears from the severity of the pain I was still experiencing. Dr Patrick immediately performed spine adjustments and manipulations of which I felt immediate relief. I continued to see Dr. Patrick three (3) times a week and each day I became stronger with less pain. I was sitting, standing, and walking again on my own and enjoying my quality of life again! However, I was not able to continue recommended maintenance visits due to insurance policy demanding that I seek physical therapy instead of chiropractic care.

Thus, I was forced to go through physical therapy from September through December 2016. The therapy however was not as effective as the healing adjustments/spinal manipulative therapy that I received by Dr. Patrick and his team. But as fate would have it; while sitting at a red traffic light On April 21, 2017, I was abruptly rear-ended by an oncoming car. So once again, I returned to receive care from Dr. Patrick and Baker Chiropractic and Wellness Center.

I am writing this testimony in June 2017, with such appreciation for the special care and attention I have received from Dr. Patrick and his staff. I am an advocate believer of holistic healing and can say that I received such healing by following through with the recommended spine adjustments and manipulations along with other therapeutic treatments for pain management as performed and/or suggested you.

So again, a great BIG Hallelujah shout out to you Dr. Patrick and your love for people and your expertise in chiropractic healing through appropriately applied spinal and other body adjustments, manipulations, etc as deem necessary for a complete outcome of Wellness.

Thank you so much!!!

— **Narkittia D.**

. . . . .

In the spring of 2017, my back was really bothering me. Several friends told me I should go see a chiropractor but I was not sure that was what I needed.

My back got a lot worse. By the time I decided to make an appointment at Baker Chiropractic and Wellness, I was in tears. The doctors at Baker Chiropractic and Wellness told me that they would be able to help. By the fall of this year, I was a lot better.

My back is getting better each time I go for an appointment. It has paid off to go to this chiropractor and I feel much better.

I would tell everyone that if you have back pain go to the doctors at Baker Chiropractic and Wellness.

I will be 80 in December so it is never too late to get help from the doctors here!

— **Marie D.**

I started coming to Baker Chiropractic and Wellness about one week ago. When I first came, I was a little unsure because I had never been to a chiropractor before. But the staff here made me feel very welcome. The first time I met with the doctor I was still a little unsure. However, after talking with Dr. Todd (Worthington) I felt confident he would be able to help me.

The reason I came to Baker Chiropractic and Wellness was due to a car accident. My body was sore, tight, and my lower and upper back was hurting. I had a hard time doing daily activities such as shopping and doing my laundry. I was also having trouble sleeping and getting out of bed was painful. This had been going on for a week or so.

After coming to Baker Chiropractic and Wellness I have noticed a tremendous change in the way my body feels. Both my upper and lower back pain has lessened. I have also noticed my sinuses have cleared up too.

I can tell that I'm getting better! Getting out and doing daily activities is easier. I'm also sleeping better.

I would refer anyone that I know to come to Baker Chiropractic and Wellness if they were having any kind of pain or discomfort in their back or shoulders.*

Sincerely,

— **Kimberly R.**

I grew up with my mom having the occasional back problems from a car accident in her youth. She would get treatment from a chiropractor and the only results that I ever recall observing was my mom tapping the refrigerator

magnets along her spine because the chiropractor told her magnets will help heal and put "things" back in place. So, my early impression was you go to a chiropractor only for back problems and magnets was the extent of the treatment. Little did I know...

In the fall of 2016, my mom fell down the stairs and she unknowingly injured her shoulder and neck when she held onto the banister to catch herself. Within a few months of her fall, she could barely lift her arm. Her doctor referred her to see a chiropractor. My mom did her research and she found the *"Best of the Best"* chiropractor in Cincinnati to make sure she got the best possible care. The chiropractor she found was Baker Chiropractic and Wellness on Red Bank Road.

Over the Christmas Holiday, the whole family got together to talk about how we all are and what is new, etc. During this conversation, I was giving my sister-in-law a neck and shoulder massage to work out several huge tension knots that were causing her severe pain and discomfort. Of course my mom, being the wonderful nurturer that she is, wanted to help. She shared her story with us and the progress she made at Baker Chiropractic and Wellness.

Mom told my sister-in-law that Baker Chiropractic was having this amazing holiday special. $21 to get your assessment, x-rays and your first adjustment and encouraged my sister-in-law to make an appointment for the next morning.

My sister-in-law has always had back issues. She broke her back playing competitive soccer in high school and has had sciatic issues ever since. My brother threw his back out about six months prior and still had some residual pain. So, my sister-in-law and brother went to Baker Chiropractic and Wellness the next morning, both taking advantage of the special, and came back with glowing reviews.

My sister-in-law told us how our neck is supposed to be at a 43 degree curve and that her neck was in the negatives. I immediately thought, well if her number is that bad, I know I had to be much worse, since I have horrible posture and the start of a bump on my back. My sister-in-law then showed us this diagram that lists all the things the spine affects. We start going thru the list and all our minds were blown. It was like going thru a checklist of all our aches, pains and random ailments. Therefore, with a combination of my mom, my sister-in-law and my brother saying it was worth it, my sister and I made our appointments.

I have had back pain since my junior year of high school. I was at swim practice one day and suddenly I had shooting pain up and down my spine. I went to the emergency room to see what was wrong. They did several tests and x-rays but they couldn't find anything wrong. I was told since there is nothing wrong, go home, take some ibuprofen and put some ice on it. My back was never the same. I would go through periods of it being fine and just be a dull ache, but then I would bend down, lean too far, pick-up something too heavy, sleep weird, whatever and Bing, there is the shooting pain again. I never would know what would trigger it. I would avoid anything I thought would cause it flair up especially when the ache escalated to a twinge. I knew it was agitated then and I had I to be careful.

Some of my other ailments was that I had been experiencing mysterious nerve issues in my hands. I would have random numbness in my pinky and ring fingers. They would also lock up for no apparent reason. I also suffered from self-diagnosed restless leg syndrome in my left leg. I even had unexplained tummy issues. When I would eat something, sometimes it would be fine, and then sometimes it wouldn't. I had also lost my sense of smell.

January 4, 2017 was my first appointment. It fit in quite nicely with my new year's resolution to actually start going to see doctors and get healthy. My appointment was with Dr. Todd Worthington and he was great. He really explained everything to me in detail. He not only answered all of my questions, but he answered them in layman's terms.

I was shocked to find out how messed up my back truly was. I had subluxations in 5 areas of my spine, hitting 4 of the 5 plexus and the cranial nerves. Basically, my entire nervous system was being affected. My neck was at -3 degrees instead of the 43 degrees, my lower back was over curved, my hips were uneven causing scoliosis in several places, making my spine look like it zig zags, plus disc deterioration in multiple places.

So needless to say, I was a hot mess and I had no clue. I was a little overwhelmed but Dr. Todd was very encouraging saying all of this was reversible, it wasn't some kind of final sentencing. He said with a lot of hard work and commitment, we can turn things around.

We hit the ground running with my treatment plan, I went 3 times week for 3 months. With the combination of the therapy, adjustments and the home kit, I got better. The body is a wonderful thing, it autocorrects as much as possible. But that can be a bad thing too because it is hard to tell when things are wrong. I had no idea I was so off, because feeling off was the norm for me. But once I started to get aligned and my body was being put back together correctly, I felt amazing. I have never felt so healthy and strong. I would call my normal everyday feeling was blah and sickly and I had no idea that is how I was really feeling. I thought it was fine and good. But now thanks to Dr. Todd and Baker Chiropractic I know better. I know what it feels like to really feel good.

My numbers have improved, I am now at 5 degrees on my neck, my hips have leveled out so I am not so zig zaggy, and my posture has improved, I haven't had a back flare up since my treatment started, I am down to the very dull ache and the occasional twinge if I push myself to far. I didn't get sick like I do every winter, my sense of smell has improved and I just feel healthy, like the way my body was designed to feel.

My treatment isn't finished; I still have a long way to go before I am 100%. I have had my own challenges with bump on my back and that will take time to reverse. This is in conjunction with getting my neck to 43 degrees. It has been hindered due to in my second month of treatment, I had my own tumble down a set of stairs and injured my shoulder and neck too. But I was fortunate that I had an appointment the next morning to immediately start work on my shoulder and neck. If I hadn't been going to a chiropractor, I would have ended up similar to my mom and not being able to lift my arm. So, I did a few steps back, but I never lost the momentum forward and I will continue to do so.

This has been a whole family affair for us and we are so grateful to everyone at Baker Chiropractic and Wellness who have help all of us on our journey. We are a healthier and happier family because of their knowledgeable expertise. I would recommend them to everyone.

You never know how much better things could be unless you try!

— **Katrina A.**

• • • • •

I began care at Baker Chiropractic and Wellness at the end of July 2017. I had injured my back at the beginning of July and was unable to participate in any activities like sports due to the injury.

I could not even throw a ball without feeling pain!

I received pain medication from medical doctors but that didn't help, so I decided to see a chiropractor instead to see if they could help.

I was unsure whether chiropractic care would help, but I am very happy with my decision to start care at Baker Chiropractic and Wellness.

They are all great people here and their care has helped me return to playing sports.

I highly recommend anyone with similar trouble to seek out care from Baker Chiropractic and Wellness.

– **Blake T.**

• • • • •

I started care here at Baker Chiropractic and Wellness less than three months ago.

I was living with low back pain for five years and severe neck pain from a car accident.

It was painful to ride my horse and pick-up my grandchildren.

To deal with the pain, I used Motrin and anti-inflammatory medications.

I was skeptical about chiropractic care at first. I didn't really believe in it. I thought it was just popping and moving bones.

After the care I have received at Baker Chiropractic and Wellness, I was able to take a 4-hour flight with absolutely no pain. I can also now ride my horse again for hours with no problem.

If I would not have come here, I would still be in pain.

I recommend that anyone who has back pain or neck pain like I did to come here and get evaluated.

— Colleen A.

• • • • •

I have had extreme low back pain, hip pain and leg pain for well over ten years which greatly limited my normal, day-to-day activities.

In my search for help with my pain issues, I would have done just about anything to get relief!

My many visits to a local chiropractor and physicians proved futile. I endured various scans, tests and procedures only to realize that it was a complete waste of my time and effort. I was getting worse and could not even enjoy being a Dad to my son!

It was then that a co-worker told me about Dr. Patrick Baker at Baker Chiropractic and Wellness.

My first adjustment seemed to be somewhat painful but when I stood up, I quickly realized that my long term pain was GONE! I was, and continue to be AMAZED at my ongoing progress!

No more pain when getting in and out of my vehicle. No more discomfort when sitting or driving for an extended period of time!

Now I can play with my son! My pain is gone! It really is!

Thank you Dr. Baker and staff!

You have all been God's hand extended to me!

— **Andrew S.**

· · · · ·

I would not be in the physical condition I am today without chiropractic care.

I came to Baker Chiropractic and Wellness on June 16, 2016 with pain in my lower right back and sciatic nerve. For more than 3 days, I had been in the worst pain I have ever encountered. I was totally incapacitated.

I attempted to relieve the pain with pills but had zero results. My wife and others suggested I look into chiropractic care for relief. So my wife set me up with an appointment at Baker Chiropractic and Wellness ASAP.

After only two (2) visits, I got relief from the pain! Chiropractic is the only way to go. This was the greatest decision I ever made to care for my body and mind.

I would and do recommend chiropractic care to everyone I encounter who is experiencing a health problem of any kind. You can have anyone contact me for a recommendation, it's for real!

Baker Chiropractic and Wellness is "The Place" for physical and mental betterment.

— Ron L.

• • • • •

It was in 2006 when my days of helping transport people and cargo came to a sudden halt. I was helping my elderly mother into the passenger seat of my minivan when something suddenly and painfully went wrong in my lower back.

I thought I had just pulled a muscle, so I began taking over-the-counter pain relievers to deal with the discomfort.

My decision not to seek treatment at the time of the injury led to serious consequences in the years that followed. I gave up activities that I used to enjoy, like bike riding, dancing, hiking, golfing, and DIY projects, because they caused too much pain – if not at the time of the activity then certainly in the days that followed.

I was missing days of work because I couldn't stand upright without pain shooting down my legs. It even changed my appearance. Gone were any shoes with more than a one inch heel. I could no longer reach my arms up to roll my hair because it involved arching my back. Bending and reaching to shave my legs or even tie my shoes involved careful planning to avoid falling over.

With less activity came weight gain and weaker core muscles which only added to the strain on my back. I became sedentary, avoiding any destination that involved climbing stairs. I chose restaurants based on the comfort of their seating. I shopped in stores with only one level or that had escalators. The more time I spent at the computer or watching television, the more problems

I had with my neck and shoulders, leading to numbness in my fingers.

I made a series of unsuccessful attempts to treat this condition over the years. I tried shoe inserts to support my arches and cushion the impact of walking. I used over-the-counter creams, sprays and patches to lessen the pain. Various doctors gave me spinal injections, decompression treatments, muscle relaxers, pain management advice and recommended stress reduction and stretching exercises. Some approaches helped relieve symptoms in the short term, but none lasted or improved the underlying condition.

To my great irritation, I realized that as of 2016 I had spent ten years, and who knows how much money, with no lasting improvement to show for it.

Then recently, while scrolling through social media postings, I saw an advertisement for Baker Chiropractic and Wellness. I didn't think I was a candidate for treatment, because I had been told that once arthritis sets in along the spine, nothing can be done except surgery. Figuring that I had nothing left to lose, I decided to go in for one assessment visit, preparing myself to be told that I was beyond being helped.

Well, the report I received was surprising as well as exciting!

Yes there was visible arthritis, and obvious curvatures of the spine, but the x-rays also showed that a lumbar disc had slipped out of alignment, causing the vertebrae to press on nearby nerves. Before I left that initial visit, I had received my first TLC (tender loving chiropractic) adjustment.

The relief from the all too familiar shooting pains was immediate! That weekend I did an unbelievable four loads of laundry in one day without any lower back pain. Never before had doing laundry been such a joy!

I am now converted to the benefits of chiropractic treatment!

Dr. Todd Worthington and the staff of the Red Bank Road office are positive, supportive, and focused on the well-being of every patient in their care.

I have a detailed treatment plan and at-home tools to support the progress I'm making during office visits. For the first time in a decade, I have experienced real pain relief!

Words cannot express what it feels like to have actual HOPE, not just wishes, for improved quality of life in the future!

— **Monica S.**

· · · · ·

I was experiencing intense lower back pain, especially in the morning. I was using ibuprophen regularly. The pain became so intense I was afraid my leg might give out and I would fall due to a subluxation. I decided to visit a chiropractor, in hopes of feeling better. Now I have no sharp pains and no ibuprophen. Now I can do my routine without the fear of my leg "giving out". I would recommend anyone to Dr. Worthington.

— **Sandra W.**

· · · · ·

I began seeing Dr. Worthington for lower back pain. I wanted a connection to total health and wellness. I liked Dr. Worthington's friendly attitude and his welcoming spirit. I now have decreased pain in my low back and pain relief during my pregnancy. I would recommend Dr. Worthington to any of my friends, particularly mothers, because of his likeminded approach to overall wellness and whole living.

— **Victoria S.**

I came to Baker Chiropractic and Wellness in August with pinched nerves, low back pain, sciatica, neck pain, and fibromyalgia. These problems had been going on for 4 to 5 months and prevented me from doing yoga, exercising and living my everyday life.

Prior to coming here, I had been taking over-the-counter medications to treat my symptoms but found no relief.

The chiropractic care I receive at Baker Chiropractic and Wellness is essential for me. It has relieved my pain and increased my mobility, all without having to use over-the-counter or prescription medications.

If not for Baker Chiropractic and Wellness, I would be in a lot of pain today. I definitely recommend this to anyone. The results I have seen are very promising!

– Nita P.

• • • • •

I had neck and lower back pain and have not experienced any symptoms since. It was a great experience. I'll look for referrals for you. Hope to see you soon. We're trying to have another baby, so when I get pregnant, I'll call you for adjustments (treatments). Thanks!

— Melissa C.

• • • • •

I have been living here in Ohio the past 3 years and I have seen 8 different chiropractors. I am a hard person to adjust because I have been in a few accidents that left me on 2 separate occasions unable to walk.

Not one chiropractor here has been able to "get all of me in", until I found Dr. Baker.

Dr. Baker was able to adjust my neck, middle and lower back unlike the other 8 different chiropractors!

What a great feeling! For the first time in 3 long years I could feel the difference in my body. I cannot describe how good that feeling is.

I never have a headache, my asthma is under control now, I stand up straighter and even my vision has improved.

Before chiropractic, I thought I had to live in chronic pain, now I have seen the difference in myself.

My quality of life has improved and I am grateful for it.

Sincerely,

— **Debbie P.**

· · · · ·

I came to Baker Chiropractic and Wellness in mid-April of this year with a sharp, stabbing pain in my lower back. Every move I made brought pain.

I had zero knowledge of chiropractic care, only an acquaintance at a local gym named Dr. Paul Baker. I had never seen a chiropractor before and viewed them as a kind of pain doctor.

The day before I came in I hurt myself moving mulch bags.

On my initial visit, Dr. Baker immediately reassured me that I came to the right place. X-Rays showed two serious stage 3 subluxations (interference) on my spine. One was at the lower part of my spine, at the point of my pain. The other was higher up near the top of my spine.

Dr. Baker put me on an aggressive program to remove the subluxations. My lower back pain disappeared in a week. By week 5, I felt rejuvenated, feeling much better than even before I was hurt.

Dr. Baker explained I was now getting a greater nerve supply to my head. I wondered how much better could I feel if I quit smoking? So I quit on May 24th.

Baker Chiropractic and Wellness has created a wellness environment that can help someone with weight or addiction problems.

If you want to feel better, live better, and be all you can be, let

Baker Chiropractic and Wellness evaluate you to put you on the right path. Their entire staff is dedicated to making that happen. I'll be a patient for the rest of my life!

– John M.

• • • • •

I woke up in the middle of the night and could not move because my back hurt so bad. In the morning we called an ambulance to transport me to the hospital. All they did was give me pain medicine and muscle relaxers. They kept me for five hours and sent me home.

After a few days I went to my family physician who sent me back to the hospital for an X-ray. The X-ray didn't show anything abnormal, but the doctor gave me more medication and sent me to physical therapy.

After going to physical therapy twice a week for two months I was still not getting much relief. I awoke another morning and found myself hardly being able to get out of bed. I then decided to go to Baker Chiropractic and Wellness.

When I arrived there I was in so much pain I was crying and could hardly walk. Everyone in the office was so nice and got me in to see Dr. Brock Frear right away. My scan showed that I had very bad degeneration in my neck and back. I immediately started getting therapy and adjustments 5 times a week. I also got massages 3 times a week.

After a month of these treatments I was still having pain and decided to get an MRI done. The results of that showed that I had a very bad herniated disc. I went to a back doctor who suggested I make an appointment with a surgeon. I shared this information with Dr. Brock and Dr. Baker who both told me to hang in there and they promised me with continued treatments and adjustments they could help me.

I stuck with it and I am so glad I did. I feel so much better and have gotten back to my normal lifestyle! I am now getting adjusted once a week to keep my back in good shape.

I am so thankful to all of the staff at Baker Chiropractic and Wellness for helping me to get my life back!

— **Ann D.**

• • • • •

I have been seeing Dr. Paul Baker and Dr. Garrett Knuckles for about six months now and I am very happy with the results.

For the past five years I have had extreme pain in my lower back, legs and abdomen areas. I had seen about ten doctors over that period of time in the pain management, orthopedic and other specialists trying to come up with a solution to my problem. This was a very depressing and painful path for myself as well as my family but I was finally brought to Baker Chiropractic and Wellness.

This is the first time I didn't hear surgery or medication was going to be needed. Dr. Paul and Dr. Garrett both spent time with me not just adjusting but talking to me about ways to improve my situation. For the first time I felt like someone took a real interest in my health and was trying to find a solution. I am not 100% yet but I am more than 50% better than I was six months ago.

The best part about my entire experience at Baker Chiropractic and Wellness is the actual staff. They are friendly, caring, and always courteous to my needs.

I will certainly recommend Baker Chiropractic and Wellness to my family and friends. Two thumbs up!

— **Steve C.**

• • • • •

Thank God for my son DeJuan for referring me to Dr. Paul Baker. Having more than 30 years of internalizing stress in a negative way, I've had constant pain in my neck, shoulders, left arm and low back.

Within 60 days of seeing Dr. Paul, my pain has decreased and my posture has improved tremendously.

I am also stronger mentally, spiritually and physically. I can even breathe better.

God's grace has given me the Power to take charge and control of my life. I have a better understanding and perspective of the benefits of the chiropractic profession. It has enabled me to heal emotionally and exercise better stress management.

I am feeling empowered and I am better – that's what's important.

Love You, God Bless You and glad we are Family.

— Berdina D.

• • • • •

I was suffering on and off from low back pain for approximately five years. It affected everything I did. I could barely move let alone play golf or basketball. I couldn't even go to the movies because sitting that long would put me in unbearable pain.

To treat the low back pain, I was taking medications (up to 15 ibuprofen daily!) and going to physical therapy. I quit the physical therapy because it never worked.

I was very skeptical of chiropractic care. I thought chiropractors were frauds but it was the last stop before I would have to face surgery and that's something I didn't want to do.

When I came to Baker Chiropractic and Wellness on July 2, 2015, I was ready for them to do anything to get me out of pain.

Today, the chiropractic care I have received from Dr. Kelly Duffner at Baker Chiropractic and Wellness has relieved all my back pain. I am once again able to be active. I recently participated in a golf outing and that wouldn't have been possible without my chiropractic care.

I highly recommend chiropractic care because it works! Without Baker Chiropractic and Wellness, I wouldn't be able to live my life the way I do now.

Before my chiropractic treatment, I hadn't played golf or participated in any type of exercise in years due to my back pain. As cliché as it sounds, I can honestly say that Baker Chiropractic and Wellness gave me my life back.

Thank you!

— **Bryan N.**

· · · · ·

I was having low back pain for a few months. The pain was really noticeable after exercising and working all day.

I was taking pain medications but wasn't getting any relief so I decided to try chiropractic care.

When I first came to Baker Chiropractic and

Wellness, I was skeptical at first but now I am relieved I decided to come here.

The chiropractic care I have received has allowed my body to heal and now the back pain is gone. If I wouldn't have come here, I am sure I would still be in pain.

The staff at Baker Chiropractic and Wellness is very nice and respectful! They create a solid plan to maximize the effectiveness of the treatment. They also educate you and show you exactly where your problem is and what problems people can have if they do not maintain proper alignment of their spine.

— **Justin N.**

• • • • •

I would like to thank you, Dr. Patrick Baker, for helping with not only with my ongoing back pain but for also offering a solution to my ten week battle with kidney stones.

I first sought out Dr. Baker's help because I threw out my back and could barely move. I was desperate to find relief from my pain as our family had tickets for the All-Star Game festivities. I needed to be on my feet and mobile for the entire week. The treatment I received for my back and shoulder offered relief faster than I expected and I was able to attend all of the events and I could not thank Dr. Baker and his staff enough.

Then at the beginning of September I was rushed to the Emergency Room with severe pain in my left side. The emergency room doctor said I had a 5mm kidney stone and advised me to make an appointment with an urologist but I would have to wait two weeks. The ER supplied me with pain medication and Flow-Max medicines to assist with passing the stone.

The stone did not pass in those two weeks, so the doctor suggested that I give it two more weeks to try to flush it out and if it did not pass by then I would need two rather expensive surgeries.

After the second urologist appointment, I mentioned everything I was going through to Dr. Baker at my very next back therapy session. When we were discussing the options that were presented to me and the cost of the surgeries and Cat Scans. I wasn't sure if he could offer any assistance but he was more than willing to listen when in reality "I was just hoping he could do something to help".

Dr. Baker said there was a kidney stone supplement pill that might be able to help in lieu of the expensive alternatives. I figured what I had nothing to lose, as my trust in Dr. Baker was growing with every visit.

I followed the directions with the supplement taking one week's worth and went back to the doctor and to my surprise they could no longer find the kidney stone on the x-ray. I also had a follow-up visit and they still could not find the kidney stone. I was elated.

So, Dr. Baker saved me from having two surgeries, the cost of the hospital stay, follow up visits and any further doctor visits. The CT scan at the ER alone was $3,186.00, so I can only imagine how much two surgeries would have cost.

I can't thank Dr. Baker and his staff enough for all the help they have given me. My back has felt so much better, I am able to help landscape our yard, tear down our shed and haul away the wood with my children and husband.

Thank you,

— Lori H

• • • • •

My name is Marlene and I was at the point of thinking "If this is what growing old is like, it's no fun!"

I had neck pain and back problems for 20+ years. I always felt sick and was unable to look up or turn my head.
I couldn't do things I enjoy like gardening or slow dancing. I couldn't hug anyone or turn my head to chat with someone.

I started chiropractic care as a last chance before having to undergo neck surgery. When I started to see signs of recovery with chiropractic care, I knew this was the answer and I wanted total and complete recovery.

Not only did I get mobility back with my neck and back but I found I could now lay on my right side without immediate dizziness.

Recently, my family doctor said I had arthritis in my wrists. Oh my aching hands. Dr. Joe Fields took a look and fixed them with just one adjustment. He takes care of my wrists every week now. No more aching!

After chiropractic care at Baker Chiropractic and Wellness, I can now:

- Look up
- Hug people
- Lay down however I want without dizziness
- Turn my head from side-to-side
- Hold my head up

I also had no idea chiropractic care could fix my aching hands and in the last two weeks, I can breath with my mouth closed. No more snoring!

I got my life back. I can live because I can move!

My name is Tim and I had been struggling with headaches, lower back pain and hip problems for a few years. I was diagnosed with osteoarthritis and given pain killers for the hip pain. I eventually had both hips replaced and I couldn't do much of anything.

The chiropractic care I have received at Baker Chiropractic and Wellness gives me energy, mobility and just makes me feel better overall. I would not be able to work 12+ hour days without chiropractic care. I am also sick far less and haven't had a case of the flu since coming here.

— Marlene and Tim M.

• • • • •

I'm a 26 year-old single mother of three beautiful children. 5 year-old Myoni and 16-month old twins (born 15 weeks premature), Morgan and Madisyn.

Before we came to Baker Chiropractic and Wellness, Morgan was barely crawling at all and Madisyn was pulling herself up on things and crawling. Morgan had been going to physical therapy but was still very stiff.

After just a few visits with Dr. Brock (Frear), Morgan is now crawling for long distances and pulling herself up on things. Madisyn is currently walking steadily. They are no longer stiff and always on the go!

The twins also used to get monthly colds that lasted 2-3 weeks but now with Chiropractic care, they have not gotten sick!

Myoni and the twins would have constipation once a month, but after Dr. Brock's chiropractic care they very regular (more than I expected)!

I was in so much pain before starting my care at Baker

Chiropractic and Wellness. Lower, middle, and upper back pain. Pain in my neck, shoulders, and Achilles. All of my pain symptoms have subsided since receiving my Chiropractic care.

I am able to resume regular activities that were very painful to do such as, laundry, working out, doing hair, and dancing!

My family and I owe our great health and able bodies to Baker Chiropractic and Dr. Brock!

— **Ronni R**

• • • • •

My name is Janice Martin and I am 62 years young. I lead a healthy lifestyle, eat close to a vegan diet, exercise on a regular basis and look physically fit, yet I have been suffering from neck, back, shoulder and leg pain for over 25 years.

Before coming to see Dr. Patrick Baker, the pain in my mid-back and lower back was becoming unbearable; I could not sit in any chair for more than a few minutes. Sleeping was not any better. When I got out of bed in the morning, I could not straighten- up for several minutes. My left leg was also radiating with pain from my groin down to my ankle. I was never comfortable.

To give some background; I was born with a dislocated hip and was positioned different ways in a body cast during the first year and a half of my life.   Because of this my left leg always turned inward.   I think this along with stress, excessive weight-bearing and lifting, (especially when I helped care for my invalid mother), caused my whole spine to become misaligned

I had been seeing another chiropractor for many years and he did give me some "relief therapy". Over the past year though, I was coming to the realization that I was feeling much worse. There had to be another chiropractor out there who could help me?

I had asked around, but was not really satisfied with any references I received. I went on line and looked at the websites of local chiropractors. The Baker Chiropractic website was definitely the most impressive, so I called and I am so glad I did.

On my initial visit to Baker Chiropractic, they took x-rays (my previous chiropractor never did). When Dr. Baker went over the results with me I cried. My neck had no natural curve at all; my pelvis was 12 mm shorter on the left side than on the right side, the vertebrae in my lower back were close to being fused and my mid-spine showed misalignment. No wonder I was in so much pain and discomfort all the time.

Dr. Baker said I was fixable, although I found this hard to believe after seeing my x-rays. I could not take the pain any longer, so I had to put my trust in this chiropractor. A treatment plan was set up for me, which I followed as directed. I started treatment in July and began feeling relief after just a few adjustments. Within 3 months I was feeling better than I had felt in 25 years! The pain that radiated down my left leg was gone. I was able to sit for much longer periods of time; I was sleeping better, and got out of bed standing straight, no more morning hunch-back. I was feeling very happy and optimistic.

It was October 26th (about 3 ½ months since I had started treatment), and I did a really stupid thing. I took my 7-year old granddaughter to a roller-skating party. I was skating around the rink like I was 12 again. I was going a little too fast, and my feet went out from under me. I landed flat on my backside. I caught myself with my hands so my head did not hit the floor and got a good whiplash too. I knew I was really hurt, but somehow managed to get myself and my granddaughter home. Within an hour I could not get off the floor. I was in excruciating pain. My son and daughter came over and wanted to take me to the emergency, but I knew what would happen in the ER and said I would wait and see Dr. Baker in the morning.

I could barely move and could not hold my head up. I had to lie in the car as my daughter drove me there. Dr. Baker took x-rays and nothing was broken, but I was misaligned worse than before I had started treatment. For 3 days I could not even hold my head up. My neck and spine had compressed and needed to decompress. Dr. Baker and his very helpful and friendly staff helped me get through this entire ordeal. They saw plenty of tears from me, but helped me to relax and heal. I went for adjustments and then home to sleep on my back with icepacks as they advised.

For 2 weeks I went for adjustments and massages, then back home to sleep and apply ice. As one part of my body would heal the pain would manifest itself in another body part; but little by little everything healed. Slowly I began to start exercising again and building myself back up with the guidance of Dr Baker and his staff. It took about 3 months, but I am finally about where I was before my accident. My recovery time was truly remarkable. If I had not been in chiropractic care, I do not know what state I would be in right now.

Baker Chiropractic is like a big family. The atmosphere is very friendly and stress-free. Everything is done in an open area so you get to interact with the staff and other patients in a relaxed and comfortable environment. I highly recommend Baker Chiropractic!

— Janice M.

• • • • •

My name is Juli Gordon and I've been receiving chiropractic care from Dr. Patrick Baker for 5 weeks. What has Dr. Patrick done for me? He has done something no other orthopedist, chiropractor, spine specialist, massage therapist, physical therapist or medication could do. He has given me back my life.

For the past 2 years, pain has robbed me from living an active lifestyle. 2 years ago, at the age of 46, I was an avid marathon runner and triathlete. Over the years I've had some back, hip, and SI joint pain, but nothing that could ever keep me from enjoying a very active lifestyle. Life isn't worth living if I can't be on the go.

Due to my own stupidity, running a marathon on an injured foot, I found myself in an air cast and crutches on and off again for about 4 months. Although my foot heeled, somehow by hobbling around in a boot, I developed excruciating lower back pain that left me completely incapacitated. Now instead of running, biking and swimming, I found myself unable to do even the simplest tasks around the house without experiencing a stabbing pain in my lower back. Turning to look out a car window, picking up heavy objects, even sitting up in bed were very painful. Sleeping became an impossible feat. I could only lay on my back, literally unable to roll to either side due to pain. The stiffness and inflammation that would build up in the nighttime would leave me barely able to get out of bed and walk in the morning. I became very unsteady on stairs. With the exception of walking, my beloved daily exercise became a thing of the past. I couldn't understand how I went from being in peak physical condition to a feeble state in a matter of months. No MRI, specialist or therapist could identify and treat the invisible bullet in my back. I sadly resigned myself to the fact that I would live with chronic pain for the rest of my life.

That all changed when I met Dr. Patrick Baker. Dr. Patrick, using the Gonstead approach to chiropractic, immediately identified the problem. He was confident, even when I wasn't, that he could restore my body and eliminate my pain. After 2 years of failed attempts by other providers, in only 5 weeks, Dr. Patrick has eliminated much of my pain and allowed me to return to a normal life. Not only can I do simple things like rolling over in bed, turning in my car, and picking up heavy items, I am now able to do intense gym workouts - performing exercises I haven't been able to do for 2 years! I'm so confident that I am on the road to recovery that I am already planning for my next, most challenging marathon yet, in just 6 months.

I am totally sold on corrective chiropractic. I will continue to do my home therapy and receive consistent chiropractic care forever. If I feel this good in only 5 weeks, I can't wait to see what's in store for me 6 months from now. I'll let everyone know how I'm feeling AFTER I finish that marathon!"

— Juli G.

• • • • •

I have had back pain since I was 13 years old. I am now 35. I went to a (medical) doctor numerous times when I was young and I was always told something different. I strained my back, I pulled a muscle, and I worked out too much. So eventually, I just stopped going to the doctor and pushed through it.

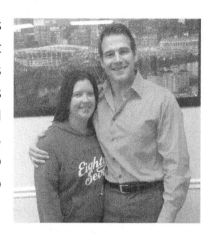

When I was young, this pain would appear and be gone within a few days, so I dealt with it. Over the years the frequency of the pain and the amount of time it took me to recover kept getting longer until December of 2012 when I hit my breaking point. I couldn't walk, stand, sleep, sit, bathe, work, or any normal things everyone does on a daily basis, without excruciating pain. On a scale from 1 to 10... I was at a 12 without moving a muscle. I landed in the ER and all they did was give me pain medications that didn't work and sent me home.

My Aunt Ann gave me the idea to call a chiropractor and I literally picked up the phone book to that section and called the first number I saw. Thankfully, the first number I dialed was Baker Chiropractic and Wellness. I started seeing Dr. Paul Baker at the

Red Bank branch and eventually started seeing Dr. Patrick Baker in Fairfield. In the beginning it was very slow going. I had so many people telling me I needed to see a medical doctor and have surgery. That was the last thing I wanted.

I had x-rays done and learned that my spine was curving in the wrong direction, in 2 places. And the lower curve was pinching my nerves causing sciatica pain in my left leg and foot. I was devastated, but the first thing Dr. Paul said was, "We can fix this. No surgery." I almost didn't believe him. But here I am. I'm walking, sitting, standing, and doing everything I couldn't a few months ago. I still have therapy ahead of me. You can't undo 20 years of damage in a few months.

I had a lot of people tell me that chiropractors don't help. That they are unreliable and I needed to see someone else. I am proof that that isn't true. I can say without a doubt, I probably wouldn't be standing today if it weren't for these wonderful people. I refer everyone I know to them. And I thank them all more than they will ever know.

— Jenny P.

• • • • •

I'm a 62 year old retired concrete man. I have been doing concrete work for 40 years with 30 years of back pain. I have had two carpal tunnel surgeries and one shoulder surgery. I do not believe in taking pain pills and will not have back surgery. My dad and brother both had back surgery and it did them no good.

My daughter was seeing Dr. Baker for back pain after having two children and she asked me to try him. I did not believe in chiropractors. I decided it could not hurt so I called. Within four weeks of three times per week visits my pain was less. After eight weeks it is almost nonexistent. I went in one day on crutches with groin pain and came out without them. I can move my neck right and left further than I have ever been able to. I did not know what it was like to live pain free again.

My sex life has doubled, which was an added bonus that makes my wife very happy. I can get down on the floor and play with my grandkids again. I can shovel snow and work on restoring my 1955 Chevy, all without pain. If something does hurt I just tell Dr. Baker and he fixes me right up. I am a happy captain now.

The staff is excellent and ready to help with anything. They work with you and your insurance. I enjoy coming in for every appointment.

I cannot describe how much better I feel. If I hadn't experienced it for myself I would never have believed it. My son is now seeing Dr. Baker for his back after he had a wreck in 1998 and broke his back. He is feeling a lot of relief already and it has only been a short amount of time for him.

I would recommend Dr. Patrick Baker and Baker Chiropractic to anyone living with any kind of chronic pain.

Thank you to Dr. Baker and all his staff.

— **Harry H.**

• • • • •

To awake in the morning and go through the entire day without a conscious thought of lower back pain, could be considered a miracle for me. Having lived with chronic back pain most of my adult life; having had two major spinal surgeries (including physical therapy) and possibly facing a third, my son Kent encouraged me to try chiropractic help from Dr. Baker before I went under the knife again.

Reluctantly, I agreed and began therapy about a year and a half ago. It was slow progress in the beginning with three visits a week. Eventually, the sessions decreased to two and finally once a week. Over the past year, I have had minor set- backs (but bounce back more quickly) mostly due to excessive exercise or long distance walking. Dr. Baker discovered that my arches were breaking down and prescribed orthotics for my walking shoes. What a difference this has made!

My quality of life has so changed!! What Dr. Baker has done to enhance and improve it is beyond words. My bucket list has increased twofold: so far this year, I bought that little red convertible (makes me feel 25 years younger), traveled on my own to locations that some can only dream about and plan to do lots more before I reach 100.

Kudos to you Dr. Baker and your team of excellent caring staff!

— J. Smith

Update to J. Smith's Story

Three Years Plus and Counting...

It has been about three years and one little red convertible later, I can actually say that I enjoy my weekly visits to Dr. Baker's office. Not only has he kept me pretty well pain free, but there has been an added perk with help with my acid reflux issue. I cannot tell you in this short testimonial how many things these doctors can help people with, all without the need for medications and/or surgeries.

Kudos again to you and your staff, Dr. Baker!

— J. Smith

· · · · ·

Update to J. Smith's Story

"Who has the courage to travel alone at the age of 76?

Here I am in East Africa on a safari. Yes, I'm 76, healthy and traveling alone.

If you had asked me that 10 years ago, I would have said, "Not me, never"!

At that time, I couldn't sit for any extended length of time, let alone fly 22 hours half way across this earth. But, with the help of Dr. Baker, my health issues are pretty much behind me.

You can see for yourself that my weekly spinal adjustments following two unsuccessful back surgeries have paid off.

I'm giving Baker Chiropractic and Wellness a big thumbs up!

Where next?

Asia or Australia are on my bucket list for 2018!"

— J. Smith

· · · · ·

Words are inadequate to express my deep gratitude and affection for the Baker Chiropractic Center family. I entered their doors with help walking because of the excruciating and debilitating pain in my back and leg. I met with Dr. Baker who immediately assured this blubbering mass of a broken person that he could help me. I was skeptical until talking with him, because three attempts with other professionals did nothing for me. I accepted his challenge and started treatment immediately, because I knew in my heart, that my healing had just begun.

After two weeks I felt like dancing (of course, I didn't – I wanted to, but didn't). I am better, not only because of the knowledgeable and aggressive treatment of Dr. Pat and Darren (my massage therapist) and the helpfulness and kindness of Jennifer, Courtney and Danielle, but also because everyone assured me that they would get me well. Their consistent and uplifting attitude was reassuring and healing. Their friendliness was endearing. I feel like part of the family.

I have also met many wonderful patients, as we share our stories with each other. My continuing treatment and rehab keeps me coming back. They will not release me until I am strong enough that this will never happen again.

I have become their greatest cheerleader; spreading the word to everyone I know who has a pain anywhere, to visit them, so they too can receive the healing that I have received over the past few weeks. Help me spread the word of this wonderful team – they are the best act in town!

I've given serious consideration to dropping their business cards and pamphlets from an airplane over Cincinnati. As of this writing, my husband has not agreed to it yet. Keep looking up!

— J. Gilman

• • • • •

I am 10 years-old. I am a gymnast and compete for the USAG Level 5 team at Cincinnati Gymnastics Academy (CGA) in Fairfield, Ohio. I started going to Doc (Patrick) Baker because I hurt my back and when I did certain skills, like my tap swings on bars or my back walkover, my lower back would hurt. My mom said that with all of the tumbling and swinging that I do during gymnastics sometimes my body needs help to get better and stay healthy.

I went to a different doctor and his help only lasted for a little while. I liked going to Doc Baker's office right away, because everyone is so nice and I get to see Ms. Krista too! After about three weeks of seeing everyone at Baker Chiropractic my back wasn't hurting nearly as bad as it was before. Every now and then it still hurt to do my back walkover though and I would go see Doc and it would feel better right away. After another couple of weeks of seeing Doc Baker I was completely pain free! He even took care of my foot when that started hurting!

My back doesn't hurt at all anymore but I still love going to see everyone at Doc Baker's office and getting my treatments and adjustments. What I think is really funny, is that a lot of parents and gymnasts from CGA go and see Doc Baker now. He makes all of us feel better!

— A. Nguyen-Storer

• • • • •

I had so many problems with back and neck that I thought there was no different feeling except hurting and aching.

I had real bad headaches and my asthma was also bad. I felt tired and had no energy.

Today, I feel like chiropractic care should be mandatory for everyone! I never knew how much difference an adjustment could make in the way I feel. I feel like a brand new woman.

Since I have been going to Dr. Paul, my headaches, back aches and other problems have disappeared. In my opinion, Dr. Paul is the best doctor around. He is caring; he explains everything before he does it.

If anyone is hurting, they should go see Dr. Paul because he can make them feel better. If he can't, he will tell them who can.

Thank you for everything. You are the best.

— **K. Bird**

• • • • •

I started seeing Dr. Paul in December 2009 after I had been experiencing chronic lower-back pain. It wasn't to the point of being debilitating but I knew it wouldn't correct itself and it was affecting my ability to run. Within a couple of weeks of therapy I was running pain-free for the first time in 14 years!

Amazed by the results I wondered if Dr. Paul could help our oldest son, Aidan, who was born with a foot deformity called metatarsus adductus. The foot specialist's plan was to put our energetic, then-3-year-old, son in a cast for 6 weeks with physical therapy to follow. We didn't want him to go through that so we thought we'd see what Dr. Paul could do. Using massage therapy and chiropractic adjustments, Aidan's foot made drastic improvement.

My wife, Carrie, also started seeing Dr. Paul for her ailments and she experienced pain relief as well. During her pregnancy with our third son, she visited Dr. Paul, which helped with discomfort she was experiencing.

Our middle son, Harrison, was getting sick quite often and the adjustments Dr. Paul performed helped his immune system.

We really appreciate the professionalism Dr. Paul and his quality staff provide while also giving each patient that personal touch. Our boys are always excited to see the Baker Chiropractic staff make themselves right at home! We feel like a part of Baker Chiropractic family and because of this, we have encouraged our friends and family members to see him.

We're so grateful for what Dr. Paul's and his staff's knowledge and expertise have been able to do for our family. Thank you so much!

— A. Kasel and Family

• • • • •

I was having low back pain and migraine headaches. I was on prescription medicine for the headaches. My back bothered me often and kept me in bed for a few days at a time.

Now I feel great thanks to Dr. Paul and Dr. Patrick Baker. I'm no longer on prescription medications for my migraines because I rarely have them anymore.

As for my lower back, it feels great too!

They are the best chiropractors and I would recommend them to anyone. Their staff makes you feel like family instead of a patient. Thank you for everything!

— **P. Bryant**

• • • • •

My name is Karen Tribby and I came to Baker Chiropractic because I was having trouble with my back and trouble walking.

I have been diagnosed with osteopina; complications from having scoliosis and TMJ in my left upper jawbone.

I went to see Dr. Patrick Baker because I noticed that he helped my co-worker, Craig Boykin with his back and walking. Craig has cerebral palsy and he has trouble with his arm being paralyzed and joints that just do not move as they should. I thought if he could help Craig, then maybe I had a chance for help.

I have been to three doctors, in the past for other medical problems and none would help including my back problems. It is very frustrating for me because when you have a serious medical problem and you hear the words, "no help", it is hard to keep you faith in doctors and people, in general. To add to my problems, I have a ventro-jugular shunt that is in my skull and I was not sure if Dr. Baker had ever heard of or worked with this type of medical procedure. I was born with hydrocephalus and this is why I have the shunt.

When I first met Dr. Patrick Baker and his staff, I noticed that they are very positive people and are committed to helping their patience's live a normal and healthy life.

I began my road to a healthier life with Baker Chiropractic in October, 2011. It has been one year now and I have had amazing results with movement returned to my back, legs, neck and shoulders. I did not realize that these areas were being affected by my back. I will continue my road to a healthier life with Baker Chiropractic as the years come. I want to live my elderly years being healthy and very active.

Thank you very much to Dr. Patrick Baker and his staff, may you continue to keep doing what you do and help people live a much healthier lifestyle.

— K. Tribby

· · · · ·

I've wanted to write my testimony since coming to Dr. Patrick Baker. I just didn't know where to start, so I'll start at the beginning. Over 35 years ago I injured my lower back at home. I went to a chiropractor (not to this one) for a brief time with no relief. Then I started working at an orthopedic office where I have been for 21 years.
One of the doctors there over the years has sent me for epidural injections, nerve blocks, physical therapy, etc. only getting temporary relief each time. The only thing that I stayed away from was pain medications and I am grateful for that. The last few years I have been getting worse, and even walking crooked. Every step was painful. I also had herniated 2 discs in my neck in 2005. Sometimes the pain would be so bad, I felt suicidal. I hadn't slept all night long in years. My husband started going to Dr. Baker when he herniated his low back. Shortly after, I had sciatica and Dr. Baker's office got me in that day. I could barely walk in, but only 1 hour later I walked out straight...and straighter than I had been in a long time! I knew right then I had found some hope! I was even able to fly to California to visit my sister. Before then, even a short car ride was painful. Every day is better. I'm even looking forward to resuming my hobbies, which are landscape photography and working in my yard. I would urge anyone who is in pain to not give up and come in to see Dr. Baker. He and his staff are wonderful! It is certainly worth it. Mere words are not

enough. And did I forget to mention, I've been going there less than 2 months! It truly will be a Merry Christmas!!

— **Carol R.**

• • • • •

Update to Carol Rice's Story

I wanted to update my testimony that I had written in December. I had only been going to Dr. Baker's 6 weeks at that time. Now it has been 4 months since I started. I continue to get better with every adjustment.

I still feel like I am dreaming sometime. I didn't think I would ever get relief from the pain.

I am sleeping great, and am able to stand and cook the great meals we are learning to eat. Before, I couldn't stand very long at a time without pain.

Dr Patrick Baker and his staff really care about their patients.

He had a seminar which was very informative. He offered a 30 day challenge and he arranged for a personal trainer 2 days a week, all at no charge to us. My husband and I have been eating the menus from one of his books for 2 weeks, along with protein powder and supplements we purchased. We can both tell a big difference! Both of our blood pressures are down.

I feel so blessed to have Dr Baker and his staff in my life. I will never forget what they have done for me. God Bless.

p.s. If this is a dream, please don't wake me!

2nd Update to Carol Rice's Story

I have been going to Dr. Patrick Baker's for 5 months now. I am currently going 2 times per week. Besides feeling better by getting maximized, I have gotten off all my meds! I got off my beta blocker, then off my cholesterol medicine. My last lab results showed everything within normal limits! Then I got off my blood pressure medicine. Since then, my blood pressure has been normal and a little lower than it was when I was on the meds.

Besides getting my spine in alignment, I have been eating better the past 6 weeks. Drinking 1 protein shake a day, no breads, pasta, sodas, snacking or eating out.

I feel so much better and I thank God that he lead me to Dr. Baker. I am sleeping better and have a better quality of life!

Thanks to Dr. Baker and all his staff for being here when I needed them.

— **Carol R.**

• • • • •

Anyone that has back pain, I can honestly tell you I understand; and those that don't cannot relate. I am physically active, run a business that is physically demanding and I thought my life was changed forever. Back surgery? Where is this going to leave me? I tried to deal with the pain, but it only got worse. My right leg started going numb, and it ached at the knee, then times at the ankle, the pain spot moved, and numbness progressed.

A customer and friend I've known for some time (Sandy) recommended Dr. Patrick and staff to my care. I was apprehensive, thought I would need back surgery for sure! Dr. Baker is truly professional and thorough; he would not touch me until he examined x-rays to know what he was dealing with. I had two bulging discs – ask Dr. Patrick where! All I wish to share with you is: don't wait! Dr. Baker and staff are chiropractic, physically and mentally healing as well; it's a great environment!

— **Don M.**

• • • • •

I've been a patient of Dr. Baker's office for about six months and since that first visit, I've made a lot of remarkable changes. I came in with constant pain in my lower back and in desperate need of help. I now have no back pain and enjoy a much healthier outlook on life. Dr. Baker said something one day that had a huge impact on my outlook. He said, "You're in a body 24 hours a day so you should feel good in it and take care of it."

That statement made me think about my health and fitness and helped sway me to join BEAT, the personal training program offered by Dr. Baker. In the five weeks since joining, I've lost 15 points and 4% body fat and feel better about life than I ever have.

Everyone in the office makes me feel welcome and important and I always leave each visit in a good mood because of the positive environment. My wife and 10-year-old daughter are now patients and I tell everyone with pain to experience the help and benefits of chiropractic care and Dr. Baker.

— Rick B.

• • • • •

I had been experiencing a nagging lower back issue for several months and the pain had reached a point at which I could no longer run (a life-long routine) or sit comfortably at work. During a conversation my neighbor Joe recommended Dr. Baker to me. Joe had been pleased with the improvement in his own back and leg pain as a result of treatments from Dr. Baker. I took Joe's recommendation and set an appointment with Dr. Baker.

After reviewing my condition Dr. Baker described the treatment plan he would be using on me and began the process of fixing the issues that years of running had created. After only a few visits there was an immediate noticeable improvement and after a few weeks I was able to run comfortably again, sit without pain and felt generally better during any other activities.

Dr. Baker and his staff were always friendly, helpful and professional. I appreciated the time that Dr. Baker took to explain my spinal issues using my x-rays to point out the areas that need attention and the treatment plan that he would use.

The results were great and the positive attitude and environment that Dr. Baker and his staff create made the healing process simple and effective. I can, and have, recommended Dr. Baker and his staff to others.

There is simply no reason to put off a visit when you are experiencing pain and discomfort.

Thank you Dr. Baker.

— Tony S.

• • • • •

I was referred to Baker Chiropractic by my sister who has taken her children as babies to Drs Paul and Pat. My daughter Rachel had a back problem related to horseback riding and I was told by her pediatrician that she probably had a hairline fracture of her spine and could require surgery. The wait to get into a pediatric orthopedic doctor was 3 months. Spinal surgery for an 11 year old did not excite me at all to say the least, so I decided to put aside my personal fears of chiropractic care and trust my sister's recommendation to take Rachel to Baker Chiropractic. As it turned out, she had a pinched nerve in her back and got immediate relief from her first visit. After three visits, she had no more back pain!

I also suffered from neck pain and low back pain and after seeing Rachel's successful treatment decided to 'take the plunge'. I had a large knot on the left side of my neck which went away completely after a few weeks of treatment. My back was so stiff, Dr. Paul almost broke his wrists trying to adjust it – okay not quite, but close! Now my spine moves as independent vertebrae instead of fused sections and feels much better!

After speaking to Dr. Paul regarding my son Andrew (9 ½ years old) who has Sensory Integration Dysfunction, he convinced me they could help Andrew. The first visit for Andrew revealed that his hips were out of alignment which resulted in one leg being an inch shorter than the other. After just a few adjustments, Andrew's legs were very close to even and he has commented on how much better his hips feel. Andrew is quite certain that Dr. Paul and Pat's treatment will contribute greatly to his professional football career someday!

Finally, my husband – ever the holistic skeptic, hurt his back moving bricks in our yard. I recommended (again and again) that he get adjusted by Baker and he finally did. His low back pain was immediately relieved.

So we are now a family helped by Baker Chiropractic on a regular basis! Many thanks to Dr. Paul and Dr. Pat for their help and expertise and to my sister Carrie for her recommendation and confidence in their treatment! Thank you.

— **Cathy H.**

• • • • •

I'm Sherry, age 68 and overall my health has been very good. I count my blessings.

Several years ago I started having an aching pain in my right groin, some days were worse than others especially on rainy days, I sometimes had to use my hands to lift my right leg into the car because of the pain, then other times it wasn't even noticeable.

My doctor told me it was arthritis and I was given an anti-inflammatory medication to help alleviate the pain. I took them for several weeks but all they did was upset my stomach so I just used over the counter medications. This went on over a period of years.

In January of 2014, the aching pain became more prevalent, it was continuous throughout the day even waking me up through the night. Not only was the groin hurting but now the right hip as well. I tried all the over-the-counter medicines but nothing worked. I even began to limp as I walked, it was time to make an appointment with my primary care physician, the date was May 2014.

During that visit I explained to the doctor about the right hip hurting, the pain in the groin area, as well as the pelvic bone being sore to the touch. When the X-ray revealed no broken bones in those areas the suggested treatment was to try another pill for several weeks. I did take the prescribed pills but by July 2014 the pain in my groin hurt so bad I called the primary care physician for another appointment but this time it was suggested I'd be seen at the Physical Medicine and Rehabilitation office.

It's August 2014 now. This examination consisted of lifting my right leg up and down and to the left and right, coming back with a recommendation to get a steroid hip injection. This would take place in September 2014. The injection did seem to help but after only one month the aching pain returned to groin and to the hip area, it's now November 2014. With the holiday season going into full swing I put my discomfort on the back burner. With just a week before Christmas, we went to New York City with family members, it was there while walking the crowded streets that I experienced sharp, excruciating pain in my inner right thigh (a 10+ on a scale of 1-10).

I would be walking one moment and the next I had to grab my husband's arm to stand as the pain in my inner right thigh took my breath away. The New Year begins it's January 2015. I have an appointment with an orthopedic doctor who then orders an MRI. The diagnosis was Tendonitis and my option was to try a second Hip Flexor Tendon Injection, which I did, along with physical therapy three times a week. After the second injection failed to stop the sharp pain, I continued going to physical therapy however it's now the end of February 2015 and whenever I turn the wrong way or step in a certain direction the pain was still there. I was losing hope that I'd ever be well again.

Now I must have a guardian angel because my neighbor Janice and I have lived next to each other for ten years. We've done yoga together, we went to various "Y" classes together and we're involved in our neighborhood ladies group "The Chick Clique". During a conversation one day, she mentions a book written by Dr. Patrick Baker, her chiropractor, and she said, "I really think he can help you Sherry".

After reading all the testimonials in that book, I began to hope that he could help me too. I thought to myself, what did I have to lose? I'd been to three doctors, had two steroid injections, taken six weeks of physical therapy and been in debilitating pain for over a year with no relief. My first visit to Dr. Baker was on Tuesday March 3, 2015 just two days after my initial phone call and I've been keeping a journal every day since then. On the second day of treatment, March 5, 2015 and only two days after reviewing my x-rays and beginning treatment on my leg, here's what I wrote:

"My leg felt lighter today, pain in groin still hurts but something's different, it feels better. I'm anxious to return for round three tomorrow".

Dr. Baker explained my problem in a way that I could understand, the adductor muscles in my right thigh were "frozen" to the pelvic bone and with certain chiropractic adjustments along with following the regiment of stretches prescribed, I would improve. Within one week (three visits) my pain went from a 10+ to a 3 and on April 25, 2015, just seven weeks and four days from my first visit with Dr. Baker, I was DANCING and I don't mean slow dancing, I was doing The Twist, The Stroll and the Electric Slide at a 50th Wedding Anniversary with no repercussions the next day!

This will be an ongoing process and it'll take time to completely heal but I can't thank you enough Dr. Baker for giving me back my life so that I could once again dance to the music!

PS: My husband Roger started seeing Dr, Baker at the same time I did back in March 2015 for sciatica pain which has affected him off and on for several years now, one time he even had to use crutches to walk around for six weeks due to the pain. Now he's a happy golfer after his visits with Dr. Baker.

Our thanks also to everyone on his staff and in the office for being so nice!

— **Sherry K.**

· · · · ·

I started visiting Dr. Garrett Knuckles at Baker Chiropractic and Wellness in late fall of 2014 due to the extreme discomfort I was experiencing in my lower back. Sometimes it was hard just to get out of bed in the morning!

My neck was also bothering me, and making my life miserable. Having these issues for over 2 years, I of course tried other chiropractors before I visited Dr. Knuckles. With little to no progress in relieving the pain, I started to think I was wasting my time.

I'm very glad I made the switch to Baker Chiropractic and Wellness, and Dr. Knuckles. None of my previous chiropractors could help me out the way Dr. Knuckles has. With regular visits to Baker, and also at-home therapy, my back issues have drastically improved. Before, I would have a hard time exercising, working in the yard or around the house, and even experienced difficulties just getting through the workday. I couldn't even enjoy my favorite hobby – playing golf.

Nowadays, I am living pain-free, and doing the things I normally do without any difficulties! Without the program Dr. Knuckles has me on, I know for certain my quality of life wouldn't be where it is today.

If I knew anyone who was experiencing back issues and general discomfort, I would do everything I could to convince them to visit Dr. Knuckles. Anyone can achieve a pain-free life with hard work, and regular visits to Baker Chiropractic ad Wellness!

Thank you Dr. Knuckles!

— **Chris F.**

• • • • •

My journey at Baker Chiropractic and Wellness began early in 2015 at the recommendation of my daughter. I must admit that I was a bit skeptical.

I came here after having lower back pain that extended down both legs for over ten years. I had been seen by several "top neurologists" who each referred me to the "next best" doctor. I had been treated with decompression surgery and medication therapy.

I saw a neurologist who told me there was nothing more that could be done and I should just continue the medication therapy. I was dependent on a cane. Extensive walking or going up and down stairs was extremely difficult.

I felt I had nothing to lose when my daughter recommended coming to Baker Chiropractic and Wellness.

After several months here, Dr. Paul (Baker) said, "You're

walking better". To be honest, I hadn't paid it much attention but now I need the cane much less and traveling up and down steps is much easier!

I recommend chiropractic care to anyone with a similar health condition. Coming to Baker Chiropractic and Wellness has made a big difference.

— Andrea J.

• • • • •

18
Bed Wetting

I wanted to give you a hearty thanks for helping Lance, my stepson, overcome his bed-wetting problem of 11 ½ years.

As you are aware, Lance was a bed-wetter 100% of the time and it was very difficult for him to cope with this problem physiologically and psychological. He is a good athlete and very social child and yet, had to deal with the problem of never being able to stay overnight at a friend's house and the problem of constantly making excuses as to why he couldn't. In addition, he always felt like something was wrong with him because he couldn't control his bladder when other children could.

But all that changed when your treatment began. First of all, Lance has immense trust and admiration for you personally. Secondly, he became fascinated with the whole treatment process and as you remember, he would ask you a great deal of questions concerning not only the treatment, but questions about the equipment and the skeletal system.

To make a long story short, today, after only a few weeks of treatment, Lance has totally conquered bed-wetting, but only with your help. He is now 100% dry and has spent the summer with his friends including at least one overnight per week. We can't thank you enough not only your professional treatment, but the positive attitude and positive responsive which you gave to our son. I would highly recommend chiropractic to anyone who is struggling with a bed-wetting problem and would be most happy to receive calls from your patients who have questions regarding our experience with solving bed-wetting.

We thank you very much for your assistance in changing Lance's life.

— J. Adams

• • • • •

Dear Dr. Joe,

In the beginning of February I started seeing you at your Madeira office. I had problems wetting the bed for several months and I had to wear pullups.

And my mom would have to wake me up to take me to the bathroom and change my bed.

Since I started seeing you, you have taken care of me and I am not wetting the bed anymore!!!!

I would tell everybody in the whole world to see you because you take care of me!!!!

Thank you!

You're the best!

— Hayley C

19
Bell's Palsy

I was diagnosed with Bell's Palsy. The entire left side of my face was paralyzed. I had difficulty blinking, smiling, speaking, eating and drinking. In addition, I had a throbbing pain in the back of my neck at the base of my skull.

I was told that I may have to wait 3-6 months for my condition to improve. As a speech pathologist, I didn't think waiting was an option.

I had never really known about chiropractic care, but with the encouragement of my husband, I figured I would give it a shot. I was ready to try anything at that point!

After just two visits at Baker Chiropractic, the neck pain was completely gone and the rate of improvement in my facial movement increased tremendously. At the end of the third week, I had regained 95% of my facial movement. I am thrilled with the results.

I feel that the chiropractic treatments allowed me to heal as completely and as rapidly as possible. I can smile again!

— M. Foster

20
Breach Baby

"My wife and I recently had our 2nd child. The baby was completely healthy and delivery couldn't have gone any smoother. We have to give a big thanks to Dr. Garrett Knuckles at Baker Chiropractic and Wellness because this was beyond our expectations.

A few months prior to the due date we found out the baby was breech transverse with spine down. The (medical) doctor informed us that this would most likely result in a high risk C-section.

I had heard Dr. Knuckles talk about the "Webster" technique and how it can help flip breeched babies. So, we crossed our fingers and my wife went in for a few adjustments.

A few weeks later and only a few days before the due date the baby flipped and the rest is history!

Thank you so much Dr. Knuckles!"*

— Nick T.

· · · · ·

Hi, My name is DJ and I am 30 weeks pregnant. I was 28 weeks pregnant when I told Dr. Patrick Baker that my baby is breach.

Dr. Patrick gave me his book (Enlightening, Adjusting and Saving Lives) to read – the section on breach babies and the adjustment he can do to help flip the baby. I read the passage in the book and the following week he adjusted me to help flip the baby.

The following day I had an ultrasound scheduled and the baby had flipped and was ready and in the right position to deliver naturally.

I definitely recommend this adjustment and I am so excited to have doc do this for me. It was a smooth and an easy adjustment. It definitely worked for me.

— DJ

· · · · ·

I came to Baker Chiropractic and Wellness for severe back pain two weeks before I was supposed to head to Germany.

I was in an accident when I was 18 and had back pain for years. I tried medications and epidurals but they didn't get rid of the pain. I couldn't walk and had pain so bad it made me cry.

After receiving treatment at Baker Chiropractic and Wellness, I was able to go on my trip to Germany and even ended up walking 30 miles while there!

When I became pregnant, the added weight shifted and again caused the pain to become severe. It interfered with my daily life and everyday functions. I couldn't even walk.

At approximately week 34-35 of my pregnancy, I found out that my baby was upside down (breach). His head was under my ribs.

I heard that the procedure by my OB to flip him was very painful and I didn't want to have that done. I came to see Dr. Baker instead.

The chiropractic adjustment was very light and wasn't painful at all. I had some Braxton-Hicks contractions and after just one treatment, I returned to my OB. The baby had already started to move. After the second treatment, he was in the right position, head down.

I would 100% recommend Baker Chiropractic and Wellness to anyone, and I often do!

I especially recommended Dr. Baker to my prenatal class.

— **Maggie O.**

• • • • •

21
Carpal Tunnel

Almost 6 months ago (March 27, 2014), I had my first meeting with Dr. Paul Baker at Baker Chiropractic and Wellness.

My symptoms were tingling and numbness in both hands and a chronically sore neck that prevented me from turning my head without pain.

May I add that I am 66 years old, in good health and am a daily athlete working-out, doing swimming, biking , running and participating in long distance triathlons and marathons.

I also work daily as a carpenter in all weather conditions throughout the year.

My fear was that my tingling hands (carpal tunnel) would prevent me from working with my hands but also keep me from riding my bike (NOT good!).

Dr. Paul assured that he would not only fix my hands but also correct a serious stenosis in my spine, improve the curvature in my neck and the slump in my shoulders and if I paid attention to the videos in his office; improve my diet.

Within a month of thrice weekly treatment I felt better. After 2 months, my numbness had subsided by 80%. By the end of 3 months, numbness was GONE.

I have continued to see Dr. Paul on a twice a week basis simply because it improves the QUALITY of my life.

I stand taller, run straighter, bike more comfortably (and faster, I have set a few personal records this race season) and my overall general health is not just good but EXCELLENT.

I would recommend to anyone to adopt a lifestyle that includes the '3 M's'

- Movement through daily exercise

- Moderation in food and drink consumption

- Manipulation (spinal adjustments) by a chiropractor.

On a closing note, I must say that I have witnessed Dr. Paul take a personal interest in his patients through humor, empathy and sincere regard for their well being that surpasses ANY health care professional that I have ever encountered.

My family including wife, son, daughter have all been the beneficiary of the corrective and preventive care of Dr. Paul's extraordinary chiropractic art.

— **Bill B.**

22
Central Canal Stenosis

Chronic pain is what compelled me to come to Baker Chiropractic and Wellness. On a scale of 1 to 10, my pain level was a 10 without question. The pain and tingling started at my hips and radiated down my legs to my toes. It prevented me from being able to do everyday housework. It stopped me from participating in one of

my favorite pastimes – golf. It got so bad that I couldn't even walk and needed to depend on a walker for any mobility whatsoever.

All this started at the beginning of the year. I originally sought the help of my medical doctor who diagnosed me as having a condition called central canal stenosis. I was prescribed medications to treat the pain which only provided temporary relief. By September, an epidural shot was recommended and that's when I felt like I needed to find a better solution. Although I was skeptical at first, I decided it was time to get help from Baker Chiropractic and Wellness.

Today, I am delighted to say that I am completely pain free! What Dr. Baker, Dr. Duffner and their wonderful team have done for me is more than any words can say! I'm back to doing everyday chores around the house and golfing with friends. If I would not have come here, I am sure I would be still be laying down in bed suffering from pain while being treated with epidurals, shots and prescription pain medications that do nothing but provide a small window of relief.

If you are battling pain, don't waste any more time and money on medications and invasive procedures that provide no long-term solution. Instead, come to Baker Chiropractic and Wellness. Find out what is causing the pain and then fix the problem. You'll find health care professionals who genuinely want to help you with a level of enthusiasm and positivity that is truly refreshing and inspiring!

— Merlanne L.

• • • • •

23
Chiari
Malformation

My 12-year-old twin girls were diagnosed with Ehlers-Danlos Syndrome (EDS) four years ago.

EDS is a group of disorders that affect connective tissues, which are tissues that support the skin, bones, blood vessels, and other organs. Defects with connective tissues cause the signs and symptoms of Ehlers-Danlos syndrome, which vary from mildly loose joints to life-threatening complications.

My girls' EDS affects their spine, legs and arms. They were having severe pain, numbness and tingling in all three areas.

Dr. Patrick Baker has been adjusting them on a regular basis and they have been using their home care kits. Their pain, numbness and tingling are decreasing.

They have been adjusted since birth. Actually, their first adjustments were at the hospital.

Shortly after birth, they were both diagnosed with Chiara Malformation, which affected their sensory and motor function. They continued with specific chiropractic adjustments and showed improvement.

The Chiara progressively got worse. So, my twins underwent decompression surgery to help improve the flow of the cerebral spinal fluid.

It's 2014 and the twins still get chiropractic adjustments. They show great benefits from having a properly aligned spine.

We will continue to receive chiropractic care for the rest of the twins' lives.

Chiropractic care has been wonderful both before and after the surgery. Many thanks to Dr. Baker and his wonderful staff!"

— **Kim S.**

24
Chronic
Aspiration

Our son, colt, was diagnosed with chronic aspiration at the age of 1 year. Along with the chronic aspiration came multiple respiratory infections, multiple doctors, multiple different medications and many other diagnoses. By the age of 2 1/2, Colt had been under general anesthesia 8 times for tests the doctors deemed medically necessary to further treat and diagnose Colt. With each test came more questions and no solutions to his problem. No doctor has ever told us why he aspirates or why he has chronic respiratory infections. The doctors are always quick to prescribe medications that they say may or may not work. What is scary to me and my husband about the medications is the horrible side effects and the long term damage the medications cause. Our frustration and disappointment were at its peak when a friend recommended Dr. Baker. We agreed to see Dr. Baker because we thought what could it hurt.

When we came to Dr. Baker's office it was a foreign environment for us. Once I got to talk to Dr. Baker and he explained chiropractic care to me, it made sense. While I was still unsure, we allowed Dr. Baker to begin adjustments on Colt. Colt was terrified in the beginning, which was to be expected, because all he has ever been able to equate doctors with is more pain. Over time Colt has grown more confident and less terrified. In fact, now he asks when he gets to see Dr. Baker again.

Colts new confidence has been wonderful but the biggest blessing we have gotten is the significant improvement in his respiratory status. He is sleeping through the night without coughing. Since we began seeing Dr. Baker he has had 1 respiratory infection, this was the only respiratory infection that didn't require steroids or breathing treatments. He was over the infection in 5 days; typically a respiratory infection for Colt lasts 2-3 weeks at minimum. Colt is now a normal, HEALTHY 3 year old who isn't taking any prescribed medications.

Dr. Baker has given us our lives back. We are truly grateful for Dr. Baker. For the first time, since Colt's health issues began, we know we are headed for success and healing. It's an indescribable feeling for parents who have spent countless sleepless nights worrying and caring for a sick child. We are firm believers in chiropractic and will recommend Dr. Baker to anyone. In fact, our other 2 children and I have started seeing Dr. Baker. We are thankful that God put Dr. Baker in our lives.

— The Hamilton Family

25
Chronic Pain

I have been living here in Ohio the past 3 years and I have seen 8 different chiropractors. I am a hard person to adjust because I have been in a few accidents that left me on 2 separate occasions unable to walk.

Not one chiropractor here has been able to "get all of me in", until I found Dr. Baker.

Dr. Baker was able to adjust my neck, middle and lower back unlike the other 8 different chiropractors!

What a great feeling! For the first time in 3 long years I could feel the difference in my body. I cannot describe how good that feeling is.

I never have a headache, my asthma is under control now, I stand up straighter and even my vision has improved.

Before chiropractic, I thought I had to live in chronic pain, now

I have seen the difference in myself.

My quality of life has improved and I am grateful for it.

Sincerely,

— **Debbie P.**

• • • • •

My name is Karen and I have been a patient of Dr. Patrick Baker for over 10 years. He has helped me through many times in my life where I was overcome with pain. Currently, he has been helping me through the pain of a fall.

I fell directly on a concrete floor after getting tangled in a dog leash. I fell flat on my backside. Hard! The pain was excruciating and I was sure I had fractured something. I went to specialists and was told nothing was fractured. Of course I received the usual pain medications and muscle relaxers but they gave me no relief. I then tried a pain specialist for steroid injections but again, no relief. They told me that I needed to do what seemed to me to be some very drastic procedures involving the nerves in my back.

This concerned me so I decided that I needed to consult with Dr. Baker. I wasn't sure if he could even help me with this particular problem but I had to try.

Dr. Baker told me he could fix me but it would take some extensive treatment. I would need to be prepared to come three days a week for several months. He said he would have to work very slowly to get my back adjusted correctly.

I had been a patient of Dr. Baker's when he worked at the Fairfield office but when he moved to the West Chester office, I felt that was just going to be too long of a drive.....but at this point I was willing to make that 75 mile drive three times a week to get better. I had faith that Dr. Baker's "anointed hands" would help me get through this pain.

So I started on this journey with Dr. Baker and he did help me. After just a few adjustments, I started to get some relief, but I still had a long way to go. There were lots of ups and downs along the way but I am finally out of pain completely!

There are no words to describe how thankful I am for the help Dr. Baker has given me. All the office staff are so helpful and uplifting. When you go to the office several times a week they become more like friends.

I tell everybody I know about Dr. Baker, Baker Chiropractic and Wellness and how they helped me through a very difficult period.

— **Karen S.**

• • • • •

Chronic pain is what compelled me to come to Baker Chiropractic and Wellness. On a scale of 1 to 10, my pain level was a 10 without question. The pain and tingling started at my hips and radiated down my legs to my toes. It prevented me from being able to do everyday housework. It stopped me from participating in one of

my favorite pastimes – golf. It got so bad that I couldn't even walk and needed to depend on a walker for any mobility whatsoever.

All this started at the beginning of the year. I originally sought the help of my medical doctor who diagnosed me as having a condition called central canal stenosis. I was prescribed medications to treat the pain which only provided temporary relief. By September, an epidural shot was recommended and that's when I felt like I needed to find a better solution. Although I was skeptical at first, I decided it was time to get help from Baker Chiropractic and Wellness.

Today, I am delighted to say that I am completely pain free! What Dr. Baker, Dr. Duffner and their wonderful team have done for me is more than any words can say! I'm back to doing everyday chores around the house and golfing with friends. If I would not have come here, I am sure I would be still be laying down in bed suffering from pain while being treated with epidurals, shots and prescription pain medications that do nothing but provide a small window of relief.

If you are battling pain, don't waste any more time and money on medications and invasive procedures that provide no long-term solution. Instead, come to Baker Chiropractic and Wellness. Find out what is causing the pain and then fix the problem. You'll find health care professionals who genuinely want to help you with a level of enthusiasm and positivity that is truly refreshing and inspiring!

— Merlanne L.

• • • • •

Bob Marley said it best when he said this quote: "Open your eyes and look within. Are you satisfied with the life you're living?"

Before coming to Baker Chiropractic and Wellness, I was not satisfied. I was miserable and I had no life. To be 27 years old and in constant pain robbed me of any joy that life had to offer me. I was taking a high dosage of pain medications daily just to take the edge off, but it never lasted. The pain just kept getting worse. I had been to 3 different chiropractors before with little success. I had since become skeptical that chiropractic could help me.

Within the first month, I definitely noticed a difference and now 4 months later I feel like a new person. I have more energy;

I stand taller, and feel better. Most importantly though I cannot stop smiling because by getting adjusted regularly by Dr. Patrick and Dr. Paul, they have given me a priceless gift. They have given me my life back, something I thought would never happen.

I have been given a new chance to live my life the way I have always dreamed I could live it. I am seeing the dreams that I thought once were dead coming back to life because my adjustments make me feel so good. I am reaching for the stars and with continuing my adjustments, I have a feeling I will capture many stars.

Thank you Dr. Patrick and Dr. Paul for changing my life and enabling me to achieve what I once thought I could never achieve.

— Jamie S.

• • • • •

As I walked into Baker Chiropractic all slumped over because of the severe pain, I was very skeptical as to what Doctors Paul and Patrick could do for me. It had, after all, been a week of misery with absolutely no relief from the prescribed prednisone.

My poor husband was desperate to get his wife back into action. He was discussing my problems to a friend, and his friend told him about Baker Chiropractic. His friend's exact words? "They're the best in the city!" Boy was he right!!"

After one visit, I was human again — far from being 100%, but I slept that night! When rehab began and Barry told me the average woman could lift 70 pounds, I was crushed. They had to take one five-pound weight OFF — I couldn't lift ANY weight now! Now, when I think back to that day (as I'm almost lifting 70 pounds), I am so grateful that this whole staff came into my life. Coming into Baker Chiropractic I feel great, as it's always a postiive and happy atmosphere. The staff and Doc Paul have always made me smile — even when I did not feel like smiling. It's been a great journey watching myself become stronger and knowing that I'm healing my back WITHOUT medicine or having to have gone through surgery.

As you're sitting there reading this, don't question for one minute if you're doing the right thing — YOU ARE!! Thanks Baker Chiropractic!

• • • • •

Several years ago after childbirth I started experiencing pelvis and back pain with popping and cracking. When I would walk I would be in extreme pain. I started seeing a chiropractor with no relief then I went to another chiropractor and still no relief. It was a chronic issue that I thought I would have to live with. Then I see a commercial about Baker Chiropractor. I knew I had to do something. The pain was unbearable.

I started seeing Dr. Baker, he gave me therapy and adjustments and he adjusted my hips, something no one else had done. At first I thought this is just another method that is not going to work. Suddenly after several weeks of adjustments I am getting relief and the pain is easing. Then I asked him about an old injury that aches all the time, it was a cracked rib that never healed properly, he treated it with therapy and adjustments and it no longer hurt. I felt he could heal everything at that point. I told him about having TMJ and the headaches that go with it, he uses a special tool and couple of appointments the headaches are gone. I got hurt playing volleyball and hurt my calf. I had it x-rayed and they said the muscle had separated from the bone and they gave me a brace and told me I needed physical therapy.

I saw Dr. Baker and he gave me physical therapy and I helped that to heal. But the worse thing that has happened to me was during a yoga class the yoga instructor was adjusting my body to a posture it could not do and something popped. I went to an orthopedic doctor who x-rayed my back and said I had three discs that were like pancakes and I had a pinched nerve in my sciatica. He referred me to a pain management doctor who gave me shots in my back to numb the area. This was very expensive and only lasted about two-week. I went to Dr. Baker and told him what happened, he has been treating my pinched nerve but he also is giving me strengthening exercises and I can honestly say I am pain free.

I recommended to all my friends and family to go and see him whether they are hurt of not but he believes in wellness and preventive methods. I feel he is my miracle worker because I thought I was going to have to live with my chronic pain the rest of my life. My husband is so thankful for all the treatment he has given me.

His office is very laid back and the girls that work there (Jennifer and Danielle) really try to get to know you and treat you like you are a part of their family. So if you are injured in any way and a doctor tells you surgery is the only option, I say go to Dr. Baker first, because sometimes there are other options and for me it is Baker Chiropractor. You have changed my life.

I just want to say thank you Dr. Patrick Baker for making me pain free. It could not have happened without you.

— **Brenda M.**

• • • • •

I choose Baker Chiropractic for two reasons, one of course is to get to the bottom of my back, neck, leg, arm, head, etc. problems. The second was to find a doctor who understands and will inform me of the science of my problems. At one time of my life I was a professional Law Librarian in NYC. Information is my bag. Information regarding my health has to make sense; medication and shots with no explanation never made sense to me. Definitely feel silly now for sticking with the drug and shot routine for so long. I am and have been a healthy person. Today, I am battling another strong woman, Mother Nature! This aging process ain't for sissy's. If you don't understand the what and why, you will die! My grandchildren are so dear to me, I want to enjoy them for a long time. Today, I have hope and no longer feel like I am turning to stone. I am so very thankful for being introduced to Baker Chiropractic.

— **Jean S.**

• • • • •

26
Colic

Sadie was born on Thanksgiving 2013 at 37 weeks. Almost immediately after bringing her home she began grunting, straining, bearing down and would turn bright red to have a bowel movement. She would do this several hours before having a bowl movement.

My husband and I would lay her on her back, bring her knees to her chest, give her tummy massage, warm baths, and even tried anal stimulation. Most of the time, this would not help. She started having difficulty eating and even sleeping, about an hour at time. She would wake up herself up straining.

We brought her to Dr. Patrick Baker at about 4 weeks old. After we came home, she had 2 bowl movements within an hour, and slept a consistent 4 hours that night!

Sadie is now 9 weeks old, she is now having normal bowl movements every morning without straining and waking herself up. The best part is she has started sleeping 6-7 hours at a time!

Mom and Dad are finally rested! Thank you Dr. Baker.

— **Emily L.**

• • • • •

My baby girl, Ellie, was born March 28, 2013, three weeks early. The first month she was having gas pains and not pooping and spitting up constantly. I took her to the Pediatrician and he said that she could go a full month without pooping, which to anyone doesn't seem logical. He said since she was early that her Sphincter needs to loosen up and that takes time. He said that he was going to put her on medicine for Acid Reflux, which I said no, as Ellie was only one month old. I immediately took her to Dr. Patrick Baker and told him the issue and he immediately said he could help with a smile on his face.

He adjusted her neck and back on a Monday afternoon. From Monday to Wednesday (the next time we saw him) she had pooped eight times and her spitting up had decreased which means Happy Mommy and Daddy.

For the first few months of her life, she saw Dr. Patrick Baker almost three times a week. Now, she goes every few weeks and is the happiest baby. I get compliments all the time for her being so happy and I always say it's because of chiropractic care. She has been sleeping through the night since she has been six weeks old, again, because of her adjustments.

A month ago, Ellie had a temperature for a few days and nothing I done would relieve it. She wouldn't sleep or eat. The Pediatrician said that she had a virus and really couldn't help. I called and talked to Dr. Brock and he came in on a Sunday to adjust her. Her fever was gone by that evening and we all got some sleep. I can't thank him enough for taking the time to come in on a weekend to help my little girl.

In closing, when we go to the office, Ellie immediately hears Dr. Patrick's or Dr. Brock's voice and smiles and giggles. She loves it there.

I just want to thank Dr. Patrick Baker, Dr. Brock, their staff and their families for the help and relief they have given my family.

— **Megan N.**

• • • • •

A few months ago my infant daughter, was having severe gas pains regularly and she wasn't pooping very often. I took her into the Pediatrician when she was 4 months old and he said that it was normal for some breastfed babies to go 7-10 days between bowel movements. Then, when she was 5 months old, I took her to another Pediatrician since the problem had not gone away and was worse. I wanted to know what I could do to alleviate her pain. The doctor said that I should start her on regular foods (which I had put off starting because of the problem) and that the problem would most likely correct itself within the next month! So, there I was with a five-month-old child who was having horrible gas pains on a daily basis and she wanted me to wait a whole month for things to get better! I was really upset because this had already been going on for quite some time and we were at a point when neither of us could take it anymore. She was in pain and so was I because I hated to hear my baby cry when I couldn't do anything to help her.

So, I asked my chiropractor, Dr. Paul Baker, if he thought he might be able to help me. He said he'd be more than happy to adjust her and he was confident he could help, so I brought her in. I was very hopeful, but didn't really know what to expect. Dr. Paul adjusted her back and neck and that night she pooped! We were thrilled because it had been so long since she had done that. I brought her in one week later and again, she pooped that night. Then she pooped the next morning and a couple more times that week. I went back each week for about 6 weeks and things just kept getting better and better. It really only took four adjustments before she was perfectly normal again. She is now a pooping machine and I couldn't be happier. She is 9 months old and as happy as can be! I can't remember the last time she had gas pains! It's a wonderful thing! I very much appreciate Dr. Paul and how great he is with my whole family and I'm grateful he was there to help me at a time when the Pediatricians didn't know what to do. It was truly an answer to our prayers.

— **Rachel**

· · · · ·

I remember the first night in the hospital after having my first child being so happy to have a healthy newborn, but he cried all night long. Everyone told me the next morning that he was just "getting used to his surroundings". The crying did not get any better after we got home, as a matter of fact it got worse. As a few weeks went on he started to cry around 11 AM, and then was fussy and crying until 4 AM. I was so exhausted and the only way I could get him to sleep was sitting in my lap on his side on a Boppy pillow. That was very unsafe, but that was the only way I could any rest. The pediatrician's said he had a horrible case of colic. He had an abdominal ultrasound, and an upper GI to see if there was anything else going on. All the tests were normal. He was on 3 different medications and none of them seemed to help. The crying then moved to the car and he cried inconsolably in the car seat. I stopped going places. It was very hard. He did not sleep through the night until the week of his first birthday. I remember it like it was yesterday. If I had only known then what I know now.

When he was 27 months old, we welcomed our daughter into the world. Everyone told me that "surely I would not have 2 kids that were that fussy, etc....this one would sleep." She didn't. When we came home from the hospital, she started to exhibit almost identical symptoms as our first. The crying started at night, then during the daytime, then in the car seat wherever I went. The big difference this time was that I had a 27 month old running around to watch after, I could not just lay down and "sleep when she slept" – which was not very often. Again, I stopped going places, it just wasn't worth it – she was screaming, then my son would start to cry because she was crying and pretty soon I was so stressed I would just go home.

When she was 4 weeks old, one of my best friends talked to Dr. Patrick about my situation and she brought me a Chiropractic magazine where he had flagged some pages for me to read. I had not experienced chiropractic care myself, let alone heard of taking children to one. I was skeptical at first and scared. I mentioned it to my husband and a few others, and they were skeptical as well and seemed to be against the idea. I went another 2 weeks with no sleep, exhausted, and not going anywhere and then had had enough. So, I made an appointment, and did not tell anyone except the babysitter who was watching my older child.

After her 5th visit, she stopped screaming in the car. She also slept for 5 hours that night. It was unbelievable. It was like this enormous weight was being lifted off my shoulders and I could live day to day again. Dr. Patrick said her neck and her lower back were really out of alignment. Since I had 2 kids that pretty much acted the same way, it makes me wonder if that was my older child's problem all along since nothing else helped him. She continued to go every week for 3 months; she was seen 22 times before Christmas and was doing great. She had turned from this unhappy, sobbing baby that would not sit a minute in the car to a happier, smiling baby. I felt like I had my life back in many ways and I of course was happier. She is now 3 and continues to go see Dr. Paul and Dr. Patrick.

Dr. Patrick and Dr. Paul have also helped me in many ways, after seeing Caroline's progress – I became a patient myself. I was later in a rear-end accident suffering from whiplash, and I went for months and was able to recuperate from that accident as well. Then while being pregnant with baby #3, I fell on the ice while carrying the dog and injured my back. Here I was pregnant, with a 4 year old, a 2 year old, and I could barely walk. I had several pinched nerves and at times I was unable to put pressure on my feet. From time to time my left leg would just give out on me and I almost fell numerous times. If it had not been for Baker Chiropractic's care during the last 3 months of my pregnancy, I don't know how I would have ever made it. I would go to my visit barely being able to walk, and when I was leaving, I walked out like a normal person. Numerous times during that time I walked into the office in absolute tears and everyone in the office was always so friendly, caring and confident.

I made it through the pregnancy and delivered a healthy baby boy. The first night in the hospital I was up all night with him. I remember crying in the hospital room, thinking "here we go again... how am I going to do this now with a 4 year old and a 2 year old?" When we got home, things did not change, and this baby cried in the car seat from day one. When he was 2 weeks old, we went to see Dr. Patrick, and sure enough, same problem as Caroline, but not as severe as hers. Within numerous visits again, he stopped crying in the car, and started to sleep. He is now 14 months old and still goes to see Dr. Patrick and Dr. Paul on a regular basis.

Words cannot describe how thankful I am to have received such fantastic care and help from Dr. Patrick and Dr. Paul during so many difficult times. They helped me through some very trying times with several of the kids and with concurrent issues with my own health. I was able to have kids that were comfortable, would sleep again and were happy. I was also able to enjoy them, rather than having them cry all the time. I wish I had known when I had my first child; I truly believe he had the same issue and the first year of his life could have been more comfortable for him if I had known to take him. I have referred many people to them as patients as I am very confident in their abilities and know they can help so many others. Everyone in the office is always so nice, friendly and welcoming. Thank you to Jennifer, Sandy and Danielle for always being so sweet and helpful in the office. And again a huge thank you to Dr. Patrick and Dr. Paul for your years of care and help and to Lana for encouraging me to make the appointment years ago. I could not have made it through all this without Baker Chiropractic's help and care.

27
Concussions

My 13 year old daughter, Brooke, experienced a potentially very serious fall, directly on the top of her head while doing a back handspring during her tumbling class.

I was watching her tumble, and as she was flipping backward in the air, she landed on her head. All of her body weight came down on her head. Obviously, we were both very scared after this incident.

Brooke was in a lot of pain and I was concerned that she had a concussion or even worse. Brooke is my only child and her health and well being are my top priority.

What I remember most, as we were walking out of the gymnasium, was feeling comforted that I could take her to be examined by Doctor Patrick. I was so grateful to know that he would be able to examine her and let me know exactly what damage had been done and what treatment she would need to hopefully make a full recovery.

By Dr. Paul Baker, Dr. Patrick Baker and Hundreds of Patients

I cannot express in words, the feeling of relief and comfort I felt when I walked into Dr. Patrick's office. I knew we were in the best hands possible. Dr. Baker immediately asked all the necessary questions and accurately assessed Brooke's injury. He treated her neck and spine and within 2 weeks she was back to 100%.

This incident caused me to realize that I have 100% trust and confidence in Dr. Patrick's judgment and skills. Considering the fact that my daughter's injury was to her head/neck/spine, getting the most accurate, expert opinion and treatment was imperative to me.

Had I been left with no other option but to take Brooke to an urgent care, I would have had doubts and concerns as to whether or not she was receiving the right care.

I realized that I have much more confidence in Dr. Baker than ANY other hospital, doctor, urgent care or specialist. I knew without the slightest of doubt, that I could fully trust Dr. Patrick with my daughter's life. This injury could have been life changing, and without knowing the severity, the only person I trusted to asses her needs was Dr. Baker.

I am so grateful to have Dr. Baker and his staff available to me to give me the peace of mind of knowing that my daughter is getting the best care possible.

— **Betsy T.**

28
Cyclic Vomiting

I began care at Baker Chiropractic and Wellness in early 2014 due to chronic headaches, migraines, and back pain. I had been plagued by headaches from the time I was a small child and chronic back pain for nearly a decade.

The migraines began roughly two years before I began my chiropractic care here. I was having between two and three migraines a week. As a mother of four children at that time, it certainly made daily life challenging. Exercise, diet and over-the-counter medications brought little relief and nothing lasting.

Shortly after receiving care at Baker Chiropractic and Wellness, I began to notice improvement. The chronic back pain had greatly diminished and within three months of starting my care, the headaches had ceased, except for the occasional stress or dehydration headache. The migraines also completely stopped with the exception of a monthly hormonal headache. Not only did I physically feel better, I felt better mentally and there was a noticeable energy increase.

I also received chiropractic care during my fifth pregnancy. Dr. Joe Fields helped my, at one point breach and at another point posterior, baby get into the right position. He also helped bring comfort to the normal pregnancy aches and is continuing to help now, six weeks postpartum, with my recovery.

I am extremely grateful for Dr. Joe and Baker Chiropractic and Wellness for their wonderful care and the gift of a healthy and more active life.

My daughter Anna also began her chiropractic care with Baker Chiropractic and Wellness in early 2014 due to headaches and cyclic vomiting syndrome.

She has dealt with headaches and cyclic vomiting from the time she was roughly two years of age. Hydration, diet modification, herbal supplementation, extra rest and over-the-counter medication offered no lasting relief. Traditional medicine can do little for cyclic vomiting, aside from treating the symptoms.

These issues greatly hindered Anna's ability to truly partake in activities that a young girl greatly enjoys. Activities such as sleepovers, camps and anything prohibiting a nap were very difficult and rare because overexertion and excitement could trigger an episode.

Once Anna began chiropractic care she experienced immediate relief from the plaguing headaches and a substantial decrease in the duration of an episode.

Now roughly a year later, Anna is almost completely free from the cyclic vomiting. Chiropractic care has greatly improved Anna's life and health, and we are forever grateful for Baker Chiropractic and Wellness and Dr. Joe Fields for their kind and tender care towards our sweet daughter.

I cannot recommend them enough, especially for the treatment of cyclic vomiting syndrome.

– Amberly W.

• • • • •

29
Degenerative Disc Disease

My name is JoAnn. My trouble began after a car wreck in high school. So this actually tells you these are long term injuries. I did wear a corrective shoe then that built my left leg up about 1 1/12 inches for two years.

As time went on years of standing in my profession took a toll on my neck and back. In the early 90's I did go see Dr. Baker got treated with success but I stopped going.

In 2004 I went for a MRI for my neck and this specialist told me surgery was not an option. The pain seemed to increase so now by 2009 I was wearing a neck brace while sleeping and got some relief.

Also in 2014 I went back to these specialists because the pain in my hip down to my right foot began to burn and felt my foot going numb. I told them about my neck injury and they said this pain was in my back and had nothing to do with my neck. (I really was not comfortable with that) They said go get an MRI and see a back surgeon right away.

Well almost 20 years later I called Dr. Baker hurting in pain. I was crying in pain and his office staff couldn't have been more compassionate.

Dr. Baker began treating me and almost immediately the pain was relieved and gone. He told me exactly step by step the plan what I needed to do and it is working! This is a journey for me but what a difference. I am not wearing my neck brace of 2 years and my pain is going away. I for the first time can see at last I am reversing what time has done to me today. Now standing straight, turning my neck, and no back pain. I have been so excited I plan to join a gym and start really concentrating on getting healthy and stronger.

I thank God for sending Dr. Baker & his staff my way and showing me so much compassion when I went there in pain and tears. I can only say to be pain free, healthy, and free from pain medications. This has been a real breakthrough for me!

Thanks again to Dr. Baker and the staff and the good Lord for using his team to help others.

God Bless you all.

— JoAnn S.

30
Degenerative
Joint Disease

My name is Janice Martin and I am 62 years young. I lead a healthy lifestyle, eat close to a vegan diet, exercise on a regular basis and look physically fit, yet I have been suffering from neck, back, shoulder and leg pain for over 25 years.

Before coming to see Dr. Patrick Baker, the pain in my mid-back and lower back becoming unbearable; I could not sit in any chair for more than a few minutes. Sleeping was not any better. When I got out of bed in the morning, I could not straighten- up for several minutes. My left leg was also radiating with pain from my groin down to my ankle. I was never comfortable.

To give some background; I was born with a dislocated hip and was positioned different ways in a body cast during the first year and a half of my life. Because of this my left leg always turned inward. I think this along with stress, excessive weight-bearing and lifting, (especially when I helped care for my invalid mother), caused my whole spine to become misaligned.

I had been seeing another chiropractor for many years and he did give me some "relief therapy". Over the past year though, I was coming to the realization that I was feeling much worse. There had to be another chiropractor out there who could help me?

I had asked around, but was not really satisfied with any references I received. I went on-line and looked at the websites of local chiropractors. The Baker Chiropractic website was definitely the most impressive, so I called and I am so glad I did.

On my initial visit to Baker Chiropractic and Wellness, they took x-rays (my previous chiropractor never did). When Dr. Baker went over the results with me I cried. My neck had no natural curve at all; my pelvis was 12 mm shorter on the left side than on the right side, the vertebrae in my lower back were close to being fused and my mid-spine showed misalignment. No wonder I was in so much pain and discomfort all the time.

Dr. Baker said I was fixable, although I found this hard to believe after seeing my x-rays. I could not take the pain any longer, so I had to put my trust in this chiropractor. A treatment plan was set up for me, which I followed as directed. I started treatment in July and began feeling relief after just a few adjustments. Within 3 months I was feeling better than I had felt in 25 years! The pain that radiated down my left leg was gone. I was able to sit for much longer periods of time; I was sleeping better, and got out of bed standing straight, no more morning hunch-back. I was feeling very happy and optimistic.

It was October 26th (about 3 ½ months since I had started treatment), and I did a really stupid thing. I took my 7-year old granddaughter to a roller-skating party. I was skating around the rink like I was 12 again. I was going a little too fast, and my feet went out from under me. I landed flat on my backside. I caught myself with my hands so my head did not hit the floor and got a good whiplash too. I knew I was really hurt, but somehow managed to get myself and my granddaughter home. Within an hour I could not get off the floor. I was in excruciating pain. My son and daughter came over and wanted to take me to the emergency, but I knew what would happen in the ER and said I would wait and see Dr. Baker in the morning.

I could barely move and could not hold my head up. I had to lie in the car as my daughter drove me there. Dr. Baker took x-rays and nothing was broken, but I was misaligned worse than before I had started treatment. For 3 days I could not even hold my head up. My neck and spine had compressed and needed to decompress. Dr. Baker and his very helpful and friendly staff helped me get through this entire ordeal. They saw plenty of tears from me, but helped me to relax and heal. I went for adjustments and then home to sleep on my back with icepacks as they advised.

For 2 weeks I went for adjustments and massages, then back home to sleep and apply ice. As one part of my body would heal the pain would manifest itself in another body part; but little by little everything healed. Slowly I began to start exercising again and building myself back up with the guidance of Dr Baker and his staff. It took about 3 months, but I am finally about where I was before my accident. My recovery time was truly remarkable.

If I had not been in chiropractic care, I do not know what state I would be in right now.

Baker Chiropractic is like a big family. The atmosphere is very friendly and stress-free.

Everything is done in an open area so you get to interact with the staff and other patients in a relaxed and comfortable environment.

I highly recommend Baker Chiropractic and Wellness!

— **Janice M.**

• • • • •

31
Depression

If it weren't for God leading me to Baker Chiropractic and Wellness, I would still be in pain and hopeless about it. I put my trust in medical doctors, and they could not help me. Much of the time, it felt like the doctors I went to didn't even believe me – passing me off as a hypochondriac – that my symptoms were "all in my head". They only gave me drugs to treat symptoms or gave me unnecessary surgeries for things that could have been helped with chiropractic care.

Although two years ago I was suffering from a long list of ailments, I came to Baker Chiropractic because I had been having debilitating pain in the back of my head and neck. I used to think my health would just get worse with time and I secretly wished I would die young because I didn't want to think about the level of pain I would be in thirty years down the road – I was already in a great deal of pain presently!

Much to my surprise, Dr. Brock Frear told me he could not only help me with my head and neck, but help me with pretty much everything else I was suffering from! Truthfully, I was skeptical at first – I had been disappointed so many times before. But the fact that he simply believed me and sympathized with me made me want to give him a chance to prove his promises.

After many reassurances, hugs, education on healthy lifestyle choices, plenty of adjustments, treatments, and home exercises – I am a new woman! Those headaches are gone, and when they occasionally try to take hold of me again, adjustments make them disappear! I have gone completely off the antidepressants I had taken for years, I have lost over thirty pounds, I no longer need cortisone shots in my knees nor suffer daily knee pain, my digestion is much improved, and currently the doctors are getting rid of my hiatal hernia! Surgeries are my last resort now, and the supplements offered at Baker Chiropractic take the place of drugs (with no side effects and better results).

The doctors at Baker Chiropractic would love to talk with you – or rather HELP you! They know they can – they have proven results! They genuinely care and are passionate about helping people. Many of them have been in dire circumstances themselves before they found how well chiropractic care works. They are like a family – waiting to adopt everyone who comes in with a desire to be physically well and bless those people with a priceless gift – hope for a brighter future. I am forever grateful to be one of those people!

— Laura K.

• • • • •

32
Developmental Problems in Children

I'm a 26 year-old single mother of three beautiful children. 5 year-old Myoni and 16-month old twins (born 15 weeks premature), Morgan and Madisyn.

Before we came to Baker Chiropractic and Wellness, Morgan was barely crawling at all and Madisyn was pulling herself up on things and crawling. Morgan had been going to physical therapy but was still very stiff.

After just a few visits with Dr. Brock (Frear), Morgan is now crawling for long distances and pulling herself up on things. Madisyn is currently walking steadily. They are no longer stiff and always on the go!

The twins also used to get monthly colds that lasted 2-3 weeks but now with Chiropractic care, they have not gotten sick!

Myoni and the twins would have constipation once a month, but after Dr. Brock's chiropractic care they very regular (more than I expected)!

I was in so much pain before starting my care at Baker Chiropractic and Wellness. Lower, middle, and upper back pain. Pain in my neck, shoulders, and Achilles. All of my pain symptoms have subsided since receiving my Chiropractic care.

I am able to resume regular activities that were very painful to do such as, laundry, working out, doing hair, and dancing!

My family and I owe our great health and able bodies to Baker Chiropractic and Dr. Brock!

— Ronni R.

• • • • •

The pregnancy with my son Billy was very stressful. My labor was induced and after more than 20 hours, he was born healthy. As a baby, he was almost on schedule with all of the normal development stages, except for his speech.

Now 6 years old, Billy was unable to focus on anything and wasn't sleeping well. There were many days where he just wouldn't cooperate with me and wouldn't get along with his siblings. His temper was high, but I thought that was typical for little boys.

Since seeing Dr. Paul Baker for the last three weeks, I have noticed several improvements with Billy. At bedtime, he no longer takes hours to fall asleep nor does he try to nap during the day. When we are doing schoolwork, he is able to sit longer and focus on his tasks. He still needs breaks if he gets overwhelmed.

I absolutely love the changes in Billy. He was always a happy and loving little guy, but now that he is on the road to better health, he is much happier. Every day he asks me if he can see Dr. Paul and get an adjustment.

Thank you to all the staff and Dr. Paul at Baker Chiropractic and Wellness

— Tracy L.

· · · · ·

I found out about Baker Chiropractic from another parent on my sons football team. The parent approached me and politely pointed out he noticed my son ran awkwardly and was one of the slowest kids on the team.

When Kasey was two, he fell and broke his femur. He was put in a body cast for two months. After the cast came off he had to learn how to sit up, crawl and walk again. I noticed right away that something wasn't right about the way he moved and that he did not like to run. We went to different medical doctors about it several times. The answer was always the same, "He will outgrow it."

Around the same time he broke his leg, he started having asthma attacks in his sleep. It was to the point I would have to run hot steamy showers to get him to stop coughing.

We also thought Kasey was a hard headed child that would not listen to anything we asked him to do. Come to find out he had so much fluid build up behind his ear drums that he could not hear us. They put tubes in his ears to drain the fluid but he continued to have ear infections at least once a month. Kasey also struggled with school work. He knew the answers to questions but was not able to process them from his mind to paper. He had a hard time blending sounds when reading simple stories.

We decided to take this parent's advice and go see Dr.

Baker. Come to find out Kasey's upper spine was out which was connected to his ears and his thinking process. His lower spine was also out from breaking his leg. Kasey has been seeing Dr. Baker for 2 years now and it is amazing the difference we see in him. He now loves to run, hasn't had a asthma attack or an ear infection in 2 years and has brought his grades up in school from needing assistance in every subject to now being above average on most subjects. Kasey is now reading chapter books and has a 100% in Math. He loves to play football, basketball and baseball. We are so proud of him.

Before we started taking him to see Dr. Baker, Kasey's self esteem was extremely low after everything he had been through. Now he is extremely happy, loves all sports and full of energy. We are very thankful for Dr. Baker and everything he has done for Kasey. I would and have recommended Dr. Baker to several friends. Thank you Dr. Baker!

— The Cook Family

• • • • •

33
Diabetic
Neuropathy

As a diabetic, I'm no stranger to pain and sickness. However, I was never prepared for the agonizing pain of diabetic neuropathy. It sneaks up on you. Starting with just a little tingle, then maybe a burning sensation. Not too bad, right? That's just how it begins. As it progresses the burning is constant, like having a match to your feet at all times until you are praying for the pain to go away. And then for the most part it does, but that's only because you've now lost all the feeling in your feet. It's like you've been walking in the snow for hours and the only sensation you can feel is pressure on your feet.

I used to consider myself to be the "Diabetic Superman". There was nothing my diabetes could do that could stop me. Neuropathy became my weakness. No matter how well adjusted or happy a person you may think you are, neuropathy will take all the joy out of your life. Want to bounce your kids on your knee? Try again, because you have daggers in your legs every time they hit your lap. It just takes all the fun out of every little thing you do, and isn't it the little things that really make us happy?

So once you realize what the problem is what do you do? If you're anything like me, you start looking for ways to "fix" the pain. I was told by every doctor I went to that there is no curing or reversing diabetic nerve damage. So what's the next step if there's no fixing it? Why narcotics of course! That's if you can find a doctor to write the prescription and don't mind being doped up all the time and developing an addiction. Not the route I wanted to take, although I did occasionally, because the pain would become unbearable. Your other alternative is "pain management".

"Pain management" is in my opinion the doctor's way of saying they can't do anything to "cure" your pain. Otherwise they would call it a "pain solution clinic". I told my doctor that I wanted any alternative to narcotics that would give me any amount of relief. You can imagine how excited I was when he told me about a new treatment called a spinal cord stimulator. It would block the signals sent by the nerves in my legs and replace them with a less painful signal. Sign me up! After more than 10 years of dealing with neuropathy this sounded like the answer to my prayers, and it was to an extent. It did indeed block the signals from my legs, but when they removed the trial stimulator I was left with excruciating pain in my back. I couldn't seem to catch a break. I didn't know if putting the actual implant in was going to leave a permanent side effect of back pain or not. Do I chance it or go on dealing with the neuropathy? To make matters worse, no doctor would admit that something was wrong with my back, despite the disc sticking out about a half inch right where my leads were put in. So after numerous MRIs, CT scans, and any other tests you can think of I felt like giving up. That's when my wife suggested I see a chiropractor. And I did.

As someone with previous experience in the medical field, I was very skeptical when I first went to see Dr. Frear at Baker Chiropractic. I don't know why? If you have heart issues you'd go to a heart doctor. So I'm not sure why I put off seeing a back doctor for back pain. Right off the bat I could tell I was going to like this place. Not only was everyone on the staff very friendly and explained the entire process to me, but how often do you see the patients happy as well? So I made my appointment, crossed my fingers and hoped he could help my back. They've done that and so much more.

After my first session, I was still sore, but by the end of the second day my back pain was completely gone. That was just the start. After every session I started to notice that I had more and more feeling in my legs and feet, something I was told would never EVER happen. So I continued to go to my appointments, and slowly but surely I'm regaining feeling in my feet. They've regained circulation and color as well.

I'm not the type of person to push any religion on anybody so I'll just leave it at this. Miracles DO happen every day. I feel like I'm proof of this. I've gone from being told that I'll never have feeling in my legs and that the lack of circulation will lead to amputation, to taking walks with my dog (and occasionally to see Dr. Brock and his staff), as well as regaining a sense of joy in my life that I never thought I would have.

I guess it pays to listen to your wife. Thank you to Dr. Brock Frear, all of his staff, and to everyone at every Baker Chiropractic office. You truly are modern day miracle workers.

— M. Shuhart

34
Ear Infections

Early one morning, I sent a message to Baker Chiropractic and Wellness. By 4:00 pm that same afternoon I started on my road to recovery.

Over 10 years ago, I began having chronic ear and sinus infections. I have 2 older sisters and they both began having ear infections around the same age. They both had PE tubes placed and never had issues with ear infections again.

My primary care doctor treated the infections for a while and then recommended that I see an Ear, Nose & Throat specialist. The first ENT told me that adults don't get chronic ear infections.

Basically, he totally blew me off. No treatment was provided!

I found another ENT and was taken seriously. Unfortunately, his interventions did not lead to success. He recommended PE tubes and they worked for about 6 months. Even with the tubes, I had 2 additional ear infections. The last ear infection resulted in the tubes being displaced. The ENT allowed my ears to "heal" and started me on an allergy medication. He also recommended that I see an allergist. I began a long road of twice a week allergy injections. The only thing that I received from the allergy injections was that I no longer have a fear of needles!

Next, the ENT recommended sinus surgery for new, more permanent PE tube placement, and to repair to my deviated septum. I would not recommend sinus surgery to anyone! It was extremely painful and took almost a month to recover from.

About a month after surgery, the ENT figured out why I was taking so long to recovery! I developed Methicillin-resistant Staphylococcus aureus (MRSA). My follow up CAT scan showed that the sinus surgery was not successful. Due to the infection, more scar tissue had formed in my nose and sinuses. His recommendation? Let's do the surgery again! I told him that I needed time to consider my options.

About 2 months later, I woke up in excruciating pain. I called my ENT and was informed that he was no longer in practice. I called my PCP and she was able to find me another ENT. The PE tubes, placed two months prior, were no longer in the place. He removed the tubes from the ear canal and told me to see him in 3 months.

My PCP finally decided that I should see a SINUS guy! I was thrilled that I would finally get relief from chronic pain and pressure. I had another CAT scan done. All my hopes were short lived. The ENT looked at my CAT scan and said that "if I was looking for surgery then I came to the wrong doctor." Surgery was the last thing on my mind. But to get relief, I would have gladly had another surgery! The doctor then recommended that I take allegra and a saline spray daily. He assured me that this would relieve all my symptoms!

A year later, he was dead wrong! In this past year alone, I have seen a doctor over 20 times! All visits were for my ears or sinuses. Even after all those visits, I still had chronic sinus pain and pressure. That pressure led to multiple ear infections in the past year.

After too many sleepless nights, I searched and found Baker Chiropractic and Wellness and submitted an appointment request at 4:00 am. I received a response from Danielle by 8:00 am with an appointment that same day. I was impressed from the moment I walked in the door. Everyone was friendly and professional. I got my first adjustment and was amazed that I had some relief. A month later, I have no ear pain! Sinuses are a work in progress but I have 100% faith that they will get better!

My x-rays showed some low back degeneration. I am a nurse and have assumed that back pain was part of the job! I am thrilled to say it is no longer part of the job! Dr. Patrick Baker is heaven sent! He provided me with a thorough understanding of the purpose of chiropractic care and what my x-rays showed. His warm, caring approach is wonderful! I cannot say enough good things about Dr. Baker and the staff at the West Chester, Ohio Chiropractic Clinic!

Their caring and compassion go beyond anything I have ever experienced! I recently experienced a death of a loved one and was overwhelmed by the support I received from Baker Chiropractic.

From a thoughtful touch to a sympathy card, Baker Chiropractic went above and beyond to share my loss. I have never had a doctor that knows so much about me and truly cares!

— Valerie H.

· · · · ·

In January, Casey failed a hearing test due to fluid that wasn't draining from both of his ears after a double ear infection in December. The doctors agreed that surgery to insert another set of tubes and remove the adenoids was the solution. While these are

both very common surgeries these days, I was still disappointed and frustrated not really understanding why this was the only solution.

Another mother told me about holistic Chiropractic care as an option and referred me to Dr. Paul Baker. She said how wonderful he was with kids. I started doing research, reading books, and found there was a connection between the spine and ear infections that had many success stories. I got Casey in as quickly as I could start treatment. I was trying not to get my hopes up, but wanted to try it before the surgery. I wasn't sure if it would work in our situation.

In the mean time, my husband asked our pediatrician about chiropractic care as an option for ear infections. While she said it was okay to try, she hadn't heard success stories about that type of treatment. Turns out Casey had a lot of compression of his spine (subluxations) right around his neck. This area does link up with the nerves that control the ears. The left ear is now completely free of fluid and the right ear (which was the worse ear) only has a little fluid left in it. We were all thrilled!

My husband, still the skeptical one, wanted another opinion and evidence that Casey's hearing was okay. I scheduled another hearing test for a week later and his hearing was absolutely normal now! I have the before and after hearing tests that document the evidence! The audiologists were very curious about what kind of things a chiropractor could do to help with fluid in the ears. I swear it was the first time they had ever heard of it.

Casey's adjustments have also helped that dreadful croupy cough he usually gets. While in Florida last week, a few of us had a cough. Casey coughed a little one morning and that was as far as it went. Usually, it would last another week to 10 days and keep him up at night. I have heard kids that get regular adjustments are healthier and have few colds that are shorter in length. With as sick as Casey has been most of his life and all the ear

infections, I can't wait! I am so sick of having all the latest cold medicines with not much relief for either of my kids.

Thanks for all your help!

— Amy D.

• • • • •

In April of 2010 I suffered from major low back pain. So much so that I had to walk bent over to be somewhat comfortable. I was referred to Doctor Baker by a fellow co-worker. I scheduled my appointment and in I went. Little did I know this would

be a life-changing event not only for me but my entire family. Besides low back pain I also suffered from dizziness, blurred vision and chronic muscle fatigue and tightness. After months of prior research I secretly believed I had MS. Well, at least that's what all the symptoms on web MD told me.

After my first visit I felt immediate relief. After only a month of adjustments at three times week and lower back exercises given by Dr. Baker's staff, my episodes of blurred vision, dizziness and muscle fatigue seemed to literally disappear. Oh yeah..... I was walking tall!

Later that year my youngest son was diagnosed with his 9th ear infection. I made Dr. Baker aware of the situation and he immediately said he could help. After several conversations with my wife she felt very uncomfortable having our nine-month old adjusted. So we were referred by his pediatrician to have tubes put in his ears. After only two weeks his ear infections were back. We hated seeing our little guy in pain. My wife finally agreed to have him evaluated by Dr. Baker. That week we brought both of our sons in. After only one adjustment his ear infection was gone. Both my sons have now been seeing Dr. Baker for several months. Still no ear infections and my six year-old has excelled drastically in his sports.

Dr. Baker not only helped my entire family regain our health, he taught me how eat clean and exercise correctly. In only four short months I lost 50lbs, 5 inches off my waist and went from 33% body fat to 18%. I also was finally able to do my first pull up of my adult life. Sad but true!

Dr. Baker is not your average Doctor. He goes above and beyond and practices what he preaches. I am glad to have found his wonderful practice. I personally feel that not only have I found the BEST doctor out there but I have also gained a great friend and mentor. I recommend him to everyone I know. I have learned that traditional medicine such as painkillers and antibiotics are NOT the answer. I believe in everything this man preaches.

Don't just make one visit and hope it helps. Continue on with his health maintenance plan and you will be a new person. I know I am!! You will enjoy every visit with him and his incredible staff. Thank you again to Baker Chiropractic!

— J. Fox

· · · · ·

My son had repeated ear infections. He had one set of tubes put in his ears and was scheduled to have a second set put in. He was getting ear infections every couple of months and the fluid wasn't draining from his ears.

Since coming to Baker Chiropractic, he hasn't had any more ear infections and hasn't needed to have the second set of tubes put in his ears.

— A. Smith

· · · · ·

189

We have been patients of Dr. Baker since August. Doc and his staff are helping us live happier, healthier lives, one adjustment at a time.

Tyler is a champion for Doc. He started to get adjustments after struggling with an ear infection for three continuous months with no relief from antibiotics. Each two week cycle the course of antibiotics became stronger, and our one-year-old boy was not getting better. When the pediatrician told me that we were looking at tubes I was determined to find something else. I happened to mention Ty's issue at Doc's one day; he gave me information on how chiropractic can help. We were desperate to find an alternative to surgery, so we decided to try it. After just three adjustments his ears were clear! Two weeks later he had a reoccurrence. This time we went straight to Doc. We decided to hold off on the antibiotics. And again, three adjustments later he was clear! This is such a relief to me as a mom, and our boy is as happy as can be!

Brian and Aubrey decided to begin seeing Doc in a proactive manner. Their bi-weekly adjustments keep them lined up and functioning in a healthy manner. We know that we will be healthier and happier if we can let our bodies work as they were designed. The staff treats each of us as real people, including our kids. Tyler is often in Krista's arms, and Danielle and Courtney let Aubrey color at the front. The office is a wonderful and comfortable environment that my kids enjoy. Ty even climbs on the table by himself at nineteen months!

We are blessed to have Dr. Baker and his staff as our doctor! Thank you for everything!

— S. Dickman

· · · · ·

My husband and I are both 25 years old with a 6 month old son. I had severe lower back pain and sciatic nerve problems that seemed to never go away. While I was pregnant, my back got worse. I did not seek chiropractic care during this time, but when my son was 8 weeks old, I couldn't take the pain anymore. Dr. Baker's office was recommended to me by family and coworkers. I decided I would try their office because I knew I didn't want any pain medicine at this young of an age.

Dr. Baker sat down with my husband, son, and me taking the time to explain the problems going on with my back. During the consultation, I was given different papers talking about chiropractic care and what they can do. At this point in time, my son had been on an antibiotic for his ear infection for about 5 days (with little to no help for his fussiness/pain). I noticed on the papers I was handed that babies can be adjusted for ear infections... so I asked about that as well. Dr. Baker explained about the adjustments he could do for our little man and how it's never good to get on

191

the "cycle of antibiotics". That night was Zeke's first adjustment. The next day, he stopped tugging at his ears. About a week later (after seeing what Doc can do), my husband was treated for his stiffness/soreness in his back and neck.

About a month into my treatment, I went to my family doctor for an ear infection. This wasn't just any normal ear infection for me. I let it go and didn't tell anyone about it until the whole side of my face hurt to physically touch. My family doctor told me the ear canal was bright red and I had a ton of fluid in my ears, and then gave me a prescription for an antibiotic. At this point in time, I was still a bit skeptical about Doc being able to help with ear infections (sorry Dr. Baker!), so I decided this would be the test. If he could help me get rid of this horrible pain/infection, I wouldn't doubt him anymore. I got adjusted right after my appointment with my family doctor. My ear/face still hurt that night, so I decided that if it still hurt the next day, I would go get the antibiotic filled and start taking it. But I didn't have to. The next morning, I woke up and the pain was almost completely gone! I was amazed! The morning after, the pain was gone. I did not have to take any antibiotics. That's when there was no doubt in my mind that Zeke not getting ear infections wasn't just coincidence. It was all about his chiropractic care!

Now, we are on maintenance care and feeling great. I don't have the pain I used to have, my husband's stiffness went away, and my son hasn't had an ear infection since (and sleeps better after being adjusted—great for us!). I can't imagine where we would be right now without the Baker Chiropractic staff. I'm sure Zeke would have had at least one set of tubes in his ears (multiple surgeries during his 6 months of life) and we would have been sore, in pain and sleep deprived at 25. We're so glad we came and got treated when we did. Thank you so much Baker staff!

— The Locke Family

35
Ehlers-Danlos
Syndrome (EDS)

"My 12-year-old twin girls were diagnosed with Ehlers-Danlos Syndrome (EDS) four years ago.

EDS is a group of disorders that affect connective tissues, which are tissues that support the skin, bones, blood vessels, and other

organs. Defects with connective tissues cause the signs and symptoms of Ehlers-Danlos syndrome, which vary from mildly loose joints to life-threatening complications.

My girls' EDS affects their spine, legs and arms. They were having severe pain, numbness and tingling in all three areas.

Dr. Patrick Baker has been adjusting them on a regular basis and they have been using their home care kits. Their pain, numbness and tingling are decreasing.

They have been adjusted since birth. Actually, their first adjustments were at the hospital. Shortly after birth, they were both diagnosed with Chiara malformation, which affected their sensory and motor function. They continued with specific chiropractic adjustments and showed improvement.

The Chiara progressively got worse. So, my twins underwent decompression surgery to help improve the flow of the cerebral spinal fluid.

It's 2014 and the twins still get chiropractic adjustments. They show great benefits from having a properly aligned spine.

We will continue to receive chiropractic care for the rest of the twins' lives.

Chiropractic care has been wonderful both before and after the surgery. Many thanks to Dr. Baker and his wonderful staff!"

— **Kim S.**

· · · · ·

36
Epilepsy

My name is Melissa, I live in Fairfield, Ohio and I'm 57 years old.

When I was 6 months old, I contracted German Measles. This developed into encephalitis and I was diagnosed with epilepsy. For many years, the doctors tried to find a medication that controlled my epilepsy. I was told I would always be taking medication for the rest of my life.

Throughout my life, I discovered many different venues that could help me to live my life as well as possible while on medication. All the different medications I had tried throughout the years have had side-effects. Before coming to see Dr. Brock,

I was doing my best to live my life as fully as possible while attempting to ameliorate the side-effects the best I could.

Prior to coming to Baker Chiropractic and Wellness, I had seen many other chiropractors for various reasons. Along the way, I picked up a lot of beneficial information. After coming to Baker Chiropractic and talking to Dr. Brock, I realized I had not been connecting the dots. Knowledge is power but power without proper implementation is fruitless.

My primary care physician had NEVER told me reduction or elimination of my medication was possible. The doctor was more than happy to keep refilling my medication month after month, year after year. I have an upcoming appointment and I look forward to the doctor's reaction! This is MY DREAM- being TOTALLY OFF my epilepsy medication PERMANENTLY!!

After only 23 visits to Baker Chiropractic, approximately 2 1/2 months (not EVEN 90 days!), I was 100% free of ALL my medication! Before talking to Dr. Brock, I had not been given any hope of EVER being off my medication.

Prior to coming here, I had been able to reduce my medication through vitamin and mineral supplementation but ELIMINATING all medication, did not seem to be a possibility. I can't tell you the number of times I have agonized over my level of care in my elderly years. "Who is going to make sure I get my medication every day?" I did not want to be a burden to anyone. I have always tried to live as healthy a lifestyle as possible but I knew there would come a day when it would no longer be in my control.

After ONLY my very FIRST visit here, I felt more energetic, more optimistic, and more vibrant! I felt like I was walking taller, like things were brighter, my attitude had improved, and I was happier! EVERY subsequent appointment, I could feel things changing. I could SEE things changing! I was VERY DEFINITELY on the right track!!

In the week following my medication elimination, my skin was smoother, my gray hair was fading, my hair was smoother and more manageable, I was thinking more clearly, sleeping soundly through the night (no getting up throughout the night), my body measurements were changing, my clothes were fitting better, and I lost FOUR POUNDS (in ONE WEEK, WITHOUT trying!) I predict 2016 will be a GREAT YEAR for me AND my family BECAUSE of the care I have received at Baker Chiropractic!

I never realized what a difference a chiropractor could make! Before coming to Baker Chiropractic and Wellness, I thought all chiropractors were the same! I was never so happy to be wrong!!

Dr. Brock and his staff have all been so helpful. Without his dedicated staff, Dr. Brock could not focus on his patients and their care, as well. Everyone has their job, what they do best and the entire office operates like a well-oiled machine! Everyone has been so positive, patient, and informative. Baker Chiropractic and Wellness for ME has been a Godsend!

I want to thank EVERYONE involved in my care now and in the future!

— Melissa N.

· · · · ·

37
Failed Back
Surgery Syndrome

To awake in the morning and go through the entire day without a conscious thought of lower back pain, could be considered a miracle for me. Having lived with chronic back pain most of my adult life; having had two major spinal surgeries (including physical therapy) and possibly facing a third, my son Kent encouraged me to try chiropractic help from Dr. Baker before I went under the knife again.

Reluctantly, I agreed and began therapy about a year and a half ago. It was slow progress in the beginning with three visits a week. Eventually, the sessions decreased to two and finally once a week. Over the past year, I have had minor set- backs (but bounce back more quickly) mostly due to excessive exercise or long distance walking. Dr. Baker discovered that my arches were breaking down and prescribed orthotics for my walking shoes. What a difference this has made!

My quality of life has so changed!! What Dr. Baker has done to enhance and improve it is beyond words. My bucket list has increased twofold: so far this year, I bought that little red convertible (makes me feel 25 years younger), traveled on my own to locations that some can only dream about and plan to do lots more before I reach 100.

Kudos to you Dr. Baker and your team of excellent caring staff!

— J. Smith

Update to J. Smith's Story

"Who has the courage to travel alone at the age of 76?

Here I am in East Africa on a safari. Yes, I'm 76, healthy and traveling alone.

If you had asked me that 10 years ago, I would have said, "Not me, never"!

At that time, I couldn't sit for any extended length of time, let alone fly 22 hours half way across this earth. But, with the help of Dr. Baker, my health issues are pretty much behind me.

You can see for yourself that my weekly spinal adjustments following two unsuccessful back surgeries have paid off.

I'm giving Baker Chiropractic and Wellness a big thumbs up!

Where next?

Asia or Australia are on my bucket list for 2018!"

— J. Smith

· · · · ·

38
Fibromyalgia

I came to Baker Chiropractic and Wellness in August with pinched nerves, low back pain, sciatica, neck pain, and fibromyalgia. These problems had been going on for 4 to 5 months and prevented me from doing yoga, exercising and living my everyday life.

Prior to coming here, I had been taking over-the-counter medications to treat my symptoms but found no relief.

The chiropractic care I receive at Baker Chiropractic and Wellness is essential for me. It has relieved my pain and increased my mobility, all without having to use over-the-counter or prescription medications.

If not for Baker Chiropractic and Wellness, I would be in a lot of pain today. I definitely recommend this to anyone. The results I have seen are very promising!

– Nita P.

. . . . .

I had fibromyalgia for approximately 7 years. When I entered the office of Baker Chiropractic for the first time, I was experiencing much pain. Especially at the base of my head, down through my neck and shoulders and all the way to my lower back. I felt like every muscle in those areas was tied into thousands of tight knots. Almost any movement caused me pain and discomfort. Many other joints in my body were hurting causing me to see many doctors in the last 7 years.

I left each of the previous doctors' offices frustrated by a lack of concern and their eagerness to prescribe medications, none of which were very effective.

After 1 ½ months of chiropractic care at Baker Chiropractic, I am a changed person. I have much less pain and tightness throughout my body. I sleep considerably better at night and therefore, have much more energy during the day. Overall, from headache to muscle and joint pain and stiffness, I just physically feel better!

Emotionally, I am much better too. I am not frustrated and better positioned to cope with issues. Baker Chiropractic understands and is knowledgeable about fibromyalgia.

It's wonderful having people be excited as I am about making me feel better!

— K. Wones

. . . . .

When I came to Dr. Patrick Baker, I was dealing with fibromyalgia, spinal misalignments, arthritis, asthma and an immune system that just wasn't fighting off things like it should. I was in constant and severe pain, fatigue, breathing problems and low energy.

Dr. Baker has greatly improved my day-to-day life. With his help, my quality of life and health are so much improved. My weekly adjustments help me function better physically. I even get through flu season much better. I was usually very ill and knocked down.

— L. Burch

. . . . .

I was suffering with fibromyalgia. I had pain and stiffness in almost all the muscles of my body. It was worse in my neck, shoulders and lower back. I also suffered from severe headaches for at least five years.

Today, my headaches are completely gone after only 4 or 5 visits. After so many years of suffering and feeling like my head was going to explode, it's such a blessing to be pain free. I don't have to take pills to make it through a day.

— D. Maxwell

. . . . .

Pain is exhausting. It becomes debilitating, it makes you irritable and it takes energy without you being aware of it. Combine pain with the side effects of cancer treatments and it becomes very difficult to find the energy and strength to handle anything.

I had multiple surgeries to treat my melanoma. As a result of these surgeries, I ended up with some nerve and muscle damage that had me in constant pain which limited my movement. I could not wear a bra due to the pain. I could not drive because I couldn't turn my head. I couldn't even lift my arms to wash my hair.

Different physicians treated me with different drugs and steroids for six months but I received minimal and short-lived relief. Not only was I disappointed in the results, I felt the source of the problem was not being addressed and my symptoms were just being treated.

Then I found Baker Chiropractic. I was skeptical at first, but I was in so much pain, it was worth a try. After two treatment sessions, a large portion of my pain was gone. I could drive again, I could sleep again and yes, I could even wear a bra again.

Dr. Baker laid out a treatment plan for me. I have been following his plan and have had a decrease in pain and an increase in motion.

— C. Schornak

· · · · ·

39
Foot Pain

I just got back from the Nike World Games in Eugene, Oregon. I thought you would like to know that I ran the 100 meters in 17 seconds. I came home with six beautiful Gold Medals thanks to the wonderful treatment I received at your office for my foot.

This is the first big event I have entered since receiving your treatment. I sincerely believe had it not been for your help, I would have not been able to run at all. No other treatment I had before I came to you had helped me.

So my heartfelt thanks to the both of you, along with your wonderful staff.

— M. Bowermaster

. . . . .

I came to Baker Chiropractic and Wellness in April 2010 after living with back pain, neck pain, shoulder pain and foot pain for approximately 2 years.

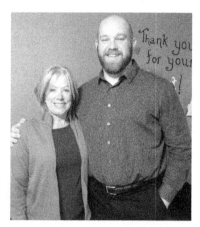

I wanted to escape the daily pain so I could simply perform my daily activities and took Advil to try and deal with it.

I was a little skeptical of chiropractic care at first but I watched a video that helped explain it. I also learned a lot from brochures about chiropractic and the Windsor Study.

Baker Chiropractic and Wellness not only got me out of pain but taught me about home care and the benefits of keeping my spine aligned.

If I would not of came here, I probably would not have been able to continue participating in the sports I love (tennis, golf, walking and weight lifting).

I definitely recommend that anyone try chiropractic care at Baker Chiropractic and Wellness. The preventative care offered to keep you away from pain and injuries is a great course of action. However, if you are already in pain, getting the source of that pain corrected is very important. Once you are out of pain, stay with chiropractic care for maintenance.

Keep up the good work!

— **Cathy S.**

40
Forward Head Posture

I decided to give chiropractic care a try in August of 2012. When I initially made the appointment to see Dr. Patrick Baker at the Fairfield Clinic of Baker Chiropractic and Wellness, I had no idea that I would still be going a year and a half later or that it would turn out to be such a life-changing decision.

I originally made the appointment because I was having severe neck pain. I could not tilt my head from side to side and I would wake up from sleeping with constant headaches. After the spinal exam and x-ray results were in, I found out that I was suffering from a condition called Forward Head Posture.

I have also suffered with migraines since I was thirteen, and Dr. Baker assured me that the chiropractic adjustments would help with those as well. I decided to proceed with Dr. Baker's treatment plan, and it was one of the best choices I have ever made.

After the first couple weeks of adjustments, I noticed a dramatic decrease in the level of neck pain I was experiencing. The constant headaches began to subside, and within a month, I was virtually pain free. And that was just the beginning. I also noticed that I was sleeping better and had more energy.

And after just a couple months of care, the migraines became less frequent. I went from having migraines three to four times a month to just three to four times a year in the time I've been a patient.

I wish I would have known years ago how much chiropractic care could help with the migraines alone. I would have started going sooner. And I urge anyone reading this that does get migraines to give it a shot. It will really improve your quality of life, much more so than those triptans we all get when we tell our doctors that we get migraines.

As if the migraine itself isn't bad enough, we're prescribed pills that only work some of the time and leave us in a sleepy haze for three days afterwards. No thanks. I'll take a massage and an adjustment instead. At least then I know I'm treating the problem and not the symptom – as evidenced by the fact that I no longer get the migraines with any real frequency. And when I do get them, they are much less severe. I no longer take triptans to treat them. Or any prescription medicine, for that matter.

Since I had been feeling so much better, I asked Dr. Baker to help me with stepping down off the antidepressant I had been prescribed three years ago because I had no lingering symptoms of depression. I felt like the meds were keeping me in a constant fog. He referred me to Dr. Theodore Cole at the Cole Center for Healing, and with their help, I was able to successfully step down off the medicine two months ago without any side effects, except a little weight loss.

Which brings me to the bonus: since attending the Baker Chiropractic Total Food Makeover seminar in February of 2013 and slowly implementing the nutrition and fitness guidelines that were provided, I have lost 40 pounds. And I'm still losing!

That's what I have enjoyed so much about this whole experience. It has been nothing but positive, and the doctors and staff are truly invested in helping you achieve your health goals. They take the time to educate you and provide you with the tools that you need to succeed. I am grateful to all of them for their help and support. I don't even want to think about what my quality of life would be like right now had I not decided to seek chiropractic care.

So if you're thinking about giving it a try, just go for it. It will be one of the best decisions you ever make.

— **Amanda G.**

41
Frozen Shoulder

For some time I have been suffering from a rotator cuff problem with my left shoulder. It finally became so debilitating that I went to orthopedic surgeons who took x-rays and an MRI. One of the surgeons recommended arthroscopic surgery.

Instead of doing that, I started physical therapy, which helped a bit, but I still had a major problem. The problem continued to worsen, and I went to a chiropractor. This also did not work and my shoulder became much worse. It was so bad that I could no longer exercise, my range of motion was severely limited and getting worse, I was unable to sleep on my shoulder, and it was waking me up every night and causing me to be very tired because of the disruption of sleep. And my shoulder was in constant pain.

Then I saw Dr. Patrick Baker when I was walking my dogs, and he asked how I was doing. When I told him of the above, he asked me to give him two weeks for a total of 6 visits. I was at this point highly skeptical and told him so. But I had nothing to lose. So I went to see Dr. Patrick at his office in West Chester, Ohio.

What Dr. Patrick accomplished in just two weeks was nothing short of miraculous to me. I am a lawyer and not prone to exaggeration or impressed easily, and I do not tell people something that is not true. I am incredibly impressed with what Dr. Patrick has done for me.

My range of motion is almost completely restored in my shoulder. I no longer have active pain. I can sleep on my shoulder, and I am again able to exercise with it. It is not yet perfect, but the improvement is dramatic. I would not have believed what he has done for me except that I have experienced it first hand. He has made a huge difference in my well-being and the quality of my life.

Thank you Dr. Patrick.

— **Tom G.**

· · · · ·

I would like to thank Dr. Patrick Baker of Baker Chiropractic and Wellness for his expedient and novel treatment of my frozen shoulder.

A frozen shoulder is extremely painful and there is very limited range of motion. This made everyday tasks very difficult and created problems for me at work. I had 2 episodes of frozen shoulder in the past and in each case the problems lasted over a year and a half. None of the health care specialists I saw were able to offer any relief.

After Dr. Baker's first treatment and a night's sleep I recovered about 60% of the range of motion. After the 3rd treatment in a week's time I had fully recovered my range of motion and had no pain.

I am deeply grateful to Dr. Patrick Baker and strongly recommend his methods for anyone suffering from frozen shoulder.

— **Paul B.**

• • • • •

42
Hand Pain and
Carpal Tunnel

I had major pain and numbness in my right hand. I could not hold anything, including a fork to feed myself. I kept on dropping things and could not feel anything at all.

I feel great now. I have 100% use of my hand and no pain or numbness. I can pick up and hold anything.

Thank you to the staff and doctors at Baker Chiropractic!

— T. Paragin

By Dr. Paul Baker, Dr. Patrick Baker and Hundreds of Patients

43
Headaches

I went from being an insurance adjuster denying chiropractic claims to becoming an advocate for chiropractic care. My migraine headaches have finally been healed after 20 years!

I was asked to see Dr. Baker by Mrs. Renee Courtney (Pitts). I was experiencing severe migraines for the last I'll say 20 years. In 1997 they were the worse I had

ever had. I was on several medicines and decided to get off them cold turkey. Of course the doctor tells you not to do this. So please don't go cold turkey. I got very ill. But to this day I do not take all that medicine any longer. I do still experience the migraines.

In 2010, I was fainting while driving and they thought I was having seizures. So the Dr. had tests ran and put me on medication even though the tests would be negative. Then I would faint sitting at my desk and now they would send me to a heart specialist and they put me on medication as well, test still negative. Every time that I would faint I would be referred to some other doctor and they would put me on a prescription and the results were endless.

I was talking to Mrs. Courtney and she asked me if I would go to Dr. Baker with her just to see what he did. I was so skeptical because I used to process claims back in the day and chiropractors were not considered doctors of health. So I was denying claims left and right.

After being there Dr. Baker told me that he could help me. Well of course this sounded great. I was impressed with the wellness care and no medicine was involved. I went for the treatment plan and was amazed how much my spine was out of line.

I started to go and to my surprise I was able to see (I mean that the pain had me all fogged up). Everything looked clearer than I could imagine. The migraine was not as severe as before. And I was heading towards improvement.

Well then Dr. Baker went on vacation. The headache came right back. You see I was not getting the treatment while he was gone. Now I can say that the adjustments I am receiving is truly helping me. I look forward to getting the adjustments and feeling better.

I only talk about what I know and I know that the adjustments really work for me. I will tell every person I know that is having pain to at least think about what the medicine is doing to your body. If you can have an adjustment and not put a foreign object in your body than take the latter.

Now it has been over a year and I feel great the headaches only comes back if I am not receiving the proper adjustments to keep my body in line.

I look forwarding to see everyone in the office. It has been an amazing journey. I love going where I can talk about the Lord and seeing what God is doing in this practice. I have seen people literally get out of wheel chairs and return to walking. Look at God operating in Dr. Baker and his practice to do his work.

Everyone at Dr. Baker's office, I would like to thank you for being so kind and helping me see that there is a better way to healthy living.

A Special Thanks to Dr. Patrick Baker (keep doing God's work).

In Christ,
— **Catherine R.**

• • • • •

I have been living here in Ohio the past 3 years and I have seen 8 different chiropractors. I am a hard person to adjust because I have been in a few accidents that left me on 2 separate occasions unable to walk.

Not one chiropractor here has been able to "get all of me in", until I found Dr. Baker.

Dr. Baker was able to adjust my neck, middle and lower back unlike the other 8 different chiropractors!

What a great feeling! For the first time in 3 long years I could feel the difference in my body. I cannot describe how good that feeling is.

I never have a headache, my asthma is under control now, I stand up straighter and even my vision has improved.

Before chiropractic, I thought I had to live in chronic pain, now I have seen the difference in myself.

My quality of life has improved and I am grateful for it.

Sincerely,

— **Debbie P.**

• • • • •

If it weren't for God leading me to Baker Chiropractic and Wellness, I would still be in pain and hopeless about it. I put my trust in medical doctors, and they could not help me. Much of the time, it felt like the doctors I went to didn't even believe me – passing me off as a hypochondriac – that my symptoms were "all in my head". They only gave me drugs to treat symptoms or gave me unnecessary surgeries for things that could have been helped with chiropractic care.

Although two years ago I was suffering from a long list of ailments, I came to Baker Chiropractic because I had been having debilitating pain in the back of my head and neck. I used to think my health would just get worse with time and I secretly wished I would die young because I didn't want to think about the level of pain I would be in thirty years down the road – I was already in a great deal of pain presently!

Much to my surprise, Dr. Brock Frear told me he could not only help me with my head and neck, but help me with pretty much everything else I was suffering from! Truthfully, I was skeptical at first – I had been disappointed so many times before. But the fact that he simply believed me and sympathized with me made me want to give him a chance to prove his promises.

After many reassurances, hugs, education on healthy lifestyle choices, plenty of adjustments, treatments, and home exercises – I am a new woman! Those headaches are gone, and when they occasionally try to take hold of me again, adjustments make them disappear! I have gone completely off the antidepressants I had taken for years, I have lost over thirty pounds, I no longer need cortisone shots in my knees nor suffer daily knee pain, my digestion is much improved, and currently the doctors are getting rid of my hiatal hernia! Surgeries are my last resort now, and the supplements offered at Baker Chiropractic take the place of drugs (with no side effects and better results).

The doctors at Baker Chiropractic would love to talk with you – or rather HELP you! They know they can – they have proven results! They genuinely care and are passionate about helping people. Many of them have been in dire circumstances themselves before they found how well chiropractic care works. They are like a family – waiting to adopt everyone who comes in with a desire to be physically well and bless those people with a priceless gift – hope for a brighter future. I am forever grateful to be one of those people!

— Laura K.

• • • • •

I was bothered by stiff necks and having a lot of trouble with neck pain and headaches. To treat my pain and discomfort I was using ice packs and taking a lot of Advil.

The stiffness and pain made it difficult to do everyday activities. I couldn't even clean my house without having to stop and lay down for awhile. I also like to golf but every time I would go golfing, I would have neck stiffness afterwards.

I put up with the pain and stiffness for over three years. I just dealt with it but I knew something needed to change. I couldn't keep living my life this way.

Prior to coming to Baker Chiropractic and Wellness, I didn't know anything about chiropractic care and how or why it works. In fact, I was very skeptical. However, after years of neck stiffness and pain, it was finally time to do something about it.

Today, I have no more neck stiffness, no more neck pain and no more headaches because of the chiropractic care I have received here. I can even go golfing now without having to deal with stiffness and discomfort.

If I would have not come to Baker Chiropractic and Wellness, I am sure I would still be dealing with the pain and not living the life I wanted to live.

Would I recommend Baker Chiropractic and Wellness to someone who is dealing with stiff necks, neck pain and headaches? Absolutely! In fact, I tell everyone about this place, how they need to learn about chiropractic care and why it can help them get out of pain.

Thank you!

— Priscilla R.

• • • • •

I was having headaches for two years or so and low back pain for over 10 years.

I knew chiropractic care could be helpful but I was never on a plan of care.

After coming to Dr. Joe Fields at Baker Chiropractic and Wellness, I no longer have the headaches.

I definitely recommend that anyone who suffers from headaches come here. If I would not have had the chiropractic care I received here, I would probably still be having the headaches today with no hope of relief.

Dr. Joe is a very thorough and compassionate doctor that effectively explains your situation, why you are having pain and his plan to correct it.

— Rhonda B.

We started going to Dr. Baker's office a couple of years ago when Olivia fell on her head and twisted her neck. After having discomfort and headaches, we decided to get her checked out. Of course, she was a mess. She started having episodes that seemed like seizures followed by a headache.

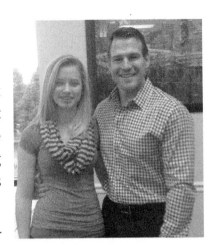

We saw many specialists. After one of her episodes, the ER said she was having hyperventilation syndrome. A cardiologist put her on an event monitor and found nothing. A hearing specialist said her ears were very healthy. An optometrist said she had healthy eyes. A neurologist said she didn't have seizures but maybe panic attacks and wanted to put her on Atenolol. An MRI showed no abnormalities.

Needless to say we were fed up with all the running around and she wasn't feeling better.

Dr. Baker's office took an x-ray showing a subluxation in her neck. Dr. Baker has been working specifically on her neck and she has been headache free.

— Julie G.

· · · · ·

I first started seeing Dr. Baker to help with my lower back. However, during my first consultation, I discussed with Dr. Baker my other issues I was having. Specifically, it was the constant headaches that had been plaguing me for months.

I had seen a few different doctors about my headaches and had multiple tests run and given a few different prescriptions. Dr. Baker explained what he thought was causing my constant headaches and the success rate that they have with headaches at Baker Chiropractic and Wellness. After a few visits, my back did not bother me anymore. More importantly, my headaches where gone.

Dr Baker was able to cure what 3 doctors including a Neurologist could not. I am a true believer in this practice and would highly recommend you talk to Dr. Baker if you have an ailment affecting you, not just back pain.

— **Robert P.**

• • • • •

I was in a boating accident 21 years ago and suffered a fractured skull and traumatic brain injury (TBI). For the last 20 years, I have been taking eight ibuprofen a day for headaches.

After the first week of adjustments by Dr. Paul Baker at Baker Chiropractic and Wellness Red Bank Clinic, I no longer had headache issues and haven't taken an ibuprofen in over a month.

This has been truly life changing for me. I can only imagine the damage all of that ibuprofen was doing to my liver, but what choice did I have? The pain and stress I was carrying around with me is gone and I feel great.

In addition, my entire body feels so much better. I have more range of motion now and the aches and pains (primarily in my lower back) that I had learned to live with are gone. Thanks Dr. Baker!

— **Greg M.**

. . . . .

I started coming to Dr. Baker due to my daily headaches that I had been having for years.

My head felt heavy and I was in constant pain. I was taking pain killers and sleeping pills prescribed by my doctor and I was also taking a minimum of 6-8 aspirins a day but nothing was helping.

Today, I am headache free. I do not have to take aspirin or any other pain relievers anymore. I am sleeping better throughout the night and don't wake up with headaches.

I feel like a new person!

— **C. Berter**

. . . . .

I suffered from migraine headaches, back pain, lack of energy and insomnia. I was taking Imitrex injections for my headaches which would provide temporary relief but they always came back.

When I came to Baker Chiropractic, the improvement started

immediately. My migraines lessened drastically, I started sleeping better, my back pain stopped and my energy level improved. I have never felt better!

Had I known how good I would feel, I would have started chiropractic treatment long ago.

— **C. Combs**

· · · · ·

I thought I was going to live the rest of my life in pain. I went from loving life to wanting to die. The pain that I had was slowly killing me.

I was taking so many pills on a daily basis to relieve my headaches and back pain. My family doctor told me this is all that could be done for me. I had gone from a bubbly, very active person, to someone I did not like at all.

I had all I could ever ask for in life - a husband, five children and a dog. I loved staying at home with my babies, working out almost every day and teaching kick boxing twice a week. I was truly blessed.

The family doctor that I trusted slowly took everything away from me. All I knew was pain, crying and no relationship with my family because I was in too much pain or too drugged up to do anything. I hated life!

That is until I walked into your office. I had no knowledge of chiropractic care. I didn't believe anyone could help me. I was amazed that my very first visit, I got relief. My all day, chronic pain was cut in half after my first adjustment. I will never forget that day. That was the day I started to get my life back.

225

My second visit to your office, I was pain free. No more pain pills. No more headaches. Being able to fall back into my old daily routine was a blessing for me.

No more screaming at my babies. No more depression. No more pills. I look in the mirror and see the person I thought was gone forever. You have healed my body and touched my heart in a way you will never know.

I am happy again. I had forgotten what that feels like. I am amazed with the knowledge you have given me. I know more about my body and my health than I ever have. I now only have one doctor and I can never thank you enough for all you have done for me.

Thank you for not only helping me but helping my children as well. No other doctor had ever seen that one of my children had one leg longer than the other. To see them become healthier and happier children is a double blessing.

If I had one wish for those who think they have to live in pain, my wish would be for them to find you. I now know we do not have to live in pain.

Thank you for all you have done and continue to do for me.

— T. Meyer

• • • • •

My 6 year old son was getting headaches at least 3 times per week. Sometimes they were so bad; he would have to go into a dark room with no noise. He would also get sick to his stomach.

I took him to an allergist, and eye doctor, and a headache specialist at Children's Hospital in Cincinnati. The specialists drugged him up so much that I no longer had my calm boy. I had one that hit himself and others, tried to be a perfectionists and threw huge fits. I demanded that he be taken off the drug Amotriptoline. They reluctantly agreed but wanted to drug him with other medications.

I was searching for help and was in tears when I approached Dr. Baker. I decided to try chiropractic care and started treatment.

Today, my son only has severe headaches once or twice a year. I am so happy to have a drug free, normal boy. He is no longer violent from medications.

As a mother, I rejoice in the fact my son no longer goes through all that pain.

— K. Faisant

· · · · ·

When I came to Dr. Baker, I had been experiencing a headache for one week. I also had soreness in my left shoulder. I was concerned because I had been taking doctor prescribed medication for my headache and it wouldn't go away.

After my very first adjustment, my headache was gone, remarkably! I also gained significant mobility.

I'm gaining a lot of knowledge about my body and how chiropractic can really change your life.

—M. Hughes

· · · · ·

My name is Amelia Aiken and I am almost 16 years old. I found out at Baker Chiropractic in February of 2009 that I have scoliosis. Before I found out that I had scoliosis, I also had allergy problems, terrible headaches, and bad migraines. My problems got worse when my little brother started acting up, but since I have been coming to Baker Chiropractic my problems have been getting better.

Dr. Baker is a miracle worker, because I thought my headaches would never go away. I found out that I also have subluxations and forward head posture. I came here first because I had an accident in the 2nd grade and it has been bothering me ever since. Since I started coming here, it has improved a lot and continues to get better every time I come to Dr. Baker. He is probably the best chiropractor anyone will have and should have. Thank you Dr. Baker!

— **Amelia**

· · · · ·

I started getting headaches and migraines when I was around 10. I have had headaches ever since. I am currently 17 and a junior in high school. Once sports start to pick up (I play year round) my neck and back pains began, which just kept getting worse until I was in pain all the time.

My headaches also were getting worse, to the point where I would have to leave school. At that point I was referred to Children's Hospital of Cincinnati Headache Clinic and was given prevention drug for headaches.

The drug, Amitriptyline HCL, worked (though I still had some major headaches) but it came with serious side effects.

I had to get off the drug so the hospital started to take me off the drug. At the same time I started going to Baker Chiropractic and Wellness. Since I have started going, I feel great emotionally and physically.

The main benefit for me is I have had a significant decrease in headaches since I started coming here!

— Tyler M.

· · · · ·

Dr. Brock Frear and Baker Chiropractic,

I just wanted to say thank you for providing such excellent care to me. Your staff members are very warm and caring as yourself.

It always surprises me as you walk thru the office you call everyone out by name and it warms my heart! "How's it going Quantessa" I feel special like family not just a patient. Thank you!

Now to the good part. I came to your chiropractic care for treatment for a back and foot injury. The last two visits I had to my primary care doctor I reported ZERO MIGRAINES – NO HEADACHES!

OMG! Please understand I had cluster migraines. Before coming to your office I was taking acute migraine tablets two or three times a week plus other pills for migraines. This was very odd to me because I have had no changes in medicine. The first month I noticed it, I stopped taking all migraine headache preventive medications which I have taken for the past 20 years. I have suffered with migraines for greater than 20 years but started nightly medication and as needed medication when the headache is coming on, plus medication for the BIG ONE – full migraine. I appreciate medication,when I found the migraine medication that worked best for me whenever I spoke to anyone that suffered with them, I tooted my horn and bragged on the medication.

Today I want to blow the trumpet so that everyone will know I HAVE NOT HAD ONEHEADACHE! No stress related migraine,no menstrual related migraine, no caffeine withdrawal related migraine..

I AM AMAZED! I never thought to seek chiropractic care for migraine relief but since I have come to you for other treatment this has been a blessing of an EXTRA BENEFIT that I have received today.

I am thankful for relief of migraine headaches and am now a friend of your chiropractic care for life. Thank you for touching my life with healing hands. I look forward to continued care because it is working for my good.

— **Quantessa G.**

. . . . .

I began care at Baker Chiropractic and Wellness in early 2014 due to chronic headaches, migraines, and back pain. I had been plagued by headaches from the time I was a small child and chronic back pain for nearly a decade.

The migraines began roughly two years before I began my chiropractic care here. I was having between two and three migraines a week. As a mother of four children at that time, it certainly made daily life challenging. Exercise, diet and over-the-counter medications brought little relief and nothing lasting.

Shortly after receiving care at Baker Chiropractic and Wellness, I began to notice improvement. The chronic back pain had greatly diminished and within three months of starting my care, the headaches had ceased, except for the occasional stress or dehydration headache. The migraines also completely stopped with the exception of a monthly hormonal headache. Not only did I physically feel better, I felt better mentally and there was a noticeable energy increase.

I also received chiropractic care during my fifth pregnancy. Dr. Joe Fields helped my, at one point breach and at another point posterior, baby get into the right position. He also helped bring comfort to the normal pregnancy aches and is continuing to help now, six weeks postpartum, with my recovery.

I am extremely grateful for Dr. Joe and Baker Chiropractic and Wellness for their wonderful care and the gift of a healthy and more active life.

My daughter Anna also began her chiropractic care with Baker Chiropractic and Wellness in early 2014 due to headaches and cyclic vomiting syndrome.

She has dealt with headaches and cyclic vomiting from the time she was roughly two years of age. Hydration, diet modification, herbal supplementation, extra rest and over-the-counter medication offered no lasting relief. Traditional medicine can do little for cyclic vomiting, aside from treating the symptoms.

These issues greatly hindered Anna's ability to truly partake in activities that a young girl greatly enjoys. Activities such as sleepovers, camps and anything prohibiting a nap were very difficult and rare because overexertion and excitement could trigger an episode.

Once Anna began chiropractic care she experienced immediate relief from the plaguing headaches and a substantial decrease in the duration of an episode.

Now roughly a year later, Anna is almost completely free from the cyclic vomiting. Chiropractic care has greatly improved Anna's life and health, and we are forever grateful for Baker Chiropractic and Wellness and Dr. Joe Fields for their kind and tender care towards our sweet daughter.

I cannot recommend them enough, especially for the treatment of cyclic vomiting syndrome.

— Amberly W.

· · · · ·

I came to Baker Chiropractic and Wellness in July of 2015. I was having really bad headaches and knots in my shoulders off and on for a couple of years.

In the five or six months prior to coming here, my headaches and knots were real bad. I was taking medicine (muscle relaxers) but not getting any long term relief. If the headaches got bad enough, I would take vicodin for them. The headaches made it really hard to focus at work. I had to look down a lot just to get a little relief.

I really didn't think about seeking chiropractic care for my headaches but my medical doctor recommended it. I also had a friend of mine from work tell me about Baker Chiropractic and Wellness.

Today, the headaches are much better after the chiropractic care I have received. I am able to focus better at work and I am not waking up in the middle of the night with severe headaches.

If I would not have come here I would probably be just be taking a lot more medications.

Baker Chiropractic and Wellness has helped me and I recommend them to others who have headaches.

This place has been great. They have a very friendly staff and operate a very organized and positive environment.

— **Ben A.**

• • • • •

44
Hearing Loss

"It was over a year ago when I noticed that I was having difficulty hearing in my right ear. The left ear was fine, but I had to turn up the volume on the TV, couldn't always hear my cell phone ringing, and was asking people to repeat themselves. I thought this was a normal aging process.

My husband was having issues with his neck and hips misaligned. He began going to Baker Chiropractic and Wellness for adjustments. They took x-rays and found exactly what areas needed to be adjusted. After he began his chiropractic visits, he insisted that I go and get X-rays too. I wasn't having any back or neck issues and didn't think I needed to go, but he insisted. So I went. The X-rays showed a serious problem with the L5 vertebrae in my lower back. Actually, I had 3.5 degeneration, the worse being 4.0, and Dr. Patrick Baker said it would take time to bring it back to normal, or at least to 2.5.

After I began the adjustments, I mentioned that I was having a problem hearing and had a ringing in my right ear. Dr. Patrick said he could correct the hearing by adjusting my atlas/axis near my ear. After 6 visits, one morning I woke up and heard a crackling sound as the ear opened up and I had no more ringing in my ear. I was so elated! It was unbelievable and so wonderful to hear clearly again! Imagine going to a chiropractor to get your hearing restored!

I continued my visits and Dr. Patrick said x-rays would be taken again after three months of adjustments. The x-rays were taken and much to my amazement, my whole body was in complete alignment. My neck was off by 9% and is now in perfect alignment, and L5 vertebrae in my lower back, which had a 3.5 degeneration was now 0%. I am now on a health maintenance plan and don't go as frequently as I did, however, I want to maintain good health and maximize my energy.

Overall, we feel much better now as our energy has been maximized. My husband is continuing his chiropractic treatments and wellness exercises and has shown much improvement having chronic sinus and neck problems. His hips are being realigned and straightened out to become even. We are staying faithful and are committed to follow the treatment plan that has been given to us by Dr. Baker.

We know you will enjoy going to the Baker Chiropractic and Wellness Center, as the environment is friendly, relaxed, and uplifting with a team of excellent, caring, and professional staff! We have been telling everyone about the amazing results we have had with Dr. Baker's expertise.

We hope you will visit the practice soon, as some of our friends are already receiving the same excellent care! God has richly blessed us through Baker Chiropractic. We highly recommend both Dr. Patrick Baker and Dr. Paul Baker to fix your problems as they have done for us. They are the best!"

— **Pauline & Ken G.**

．．．．．

In January, Casey failed a hearing test due to fluid that wasn't draining from both of his ears after a double ear infection in December. The doctors agreed that surgery to insert another set of tubes and remove the adenoids

was the solution. While these are both very common surgeries these days, I was still disappointed and frustrated not really understanding why this was the only solution.

Another mother told me about holistic Chiropractic care as an option and referred me to Dr. Paul Baker. She said how wonderful he was with kids. I started doing research, reading books, and found there was a connection between the spine and ear infections that had many success stories. I got Casey in as quickly as I could start treatment. I was trying not to get my hopes up, but wanted to try it before the surgery. I wasn't sure if it would work in our situation.

In the mean time, my husband asked our pediatrician about chiropractic care as an option for ear infections. While she said it was okay to try, she hadn't heard success stories about that type of treatment. Turns out Casey had a lot of compression of his spine (subluxations) right around his neck. This area does link up with the nerves that control the ears. The left ear is now completely free of fluid and the right ear (which was the worse ear) only has a little fluid left in it. We were all thrilled!

My husband, still the skeptical one, wanted another opinion and evidence that Casey's hearing was okay. I scheduled another hearing test for a week later and his hearing was absolutely normal now! I have the before and after hearing tests that document the evidence! The audiologists were very curious about what kind of things a chiropractor could do to help with fluid in the ears. I swear it was the first time they had ever heard of it.

Casey's adjustments have also helped that dreadful croupy cough he usually gets. While in Florida last week, a few of us had a cough. Casey coughed a little one morning and that was as far as it went. Usually, it would last another week to 10 days and keep him up at night. I have heard kids that get regular adjustments are healthier and have few colds that are shorter in length. With as sick as Casey has been most of his life and all the ear

infections, I can't wait! I am so sick of having all the latest cold medicines with not much relief for either of my kids.

Thanks for all your help!

— **Amy D.**

· · · · ·

45
Heel Pain

I came to Baker Chiropractic and Wellness about three weeks ago with severe heel pain.

I had been suffering from the heel pain for about 10 days. I couldn't play sports, coach baseball or even walk normal.

I was taking Advil and tried stretching to find some relief but nothing worked. Although I was skeptical that chiropractic care could help me, I decided to give Baker Chiropractic and Wellness a try.

Today, I have zero pain! I can play basketball again. I can coach baseball and I can walk normal.

If I would not have come to Baker Chiropractic and Wellness, I am sure I would be seeing a medical doctor and taking pain medications. I may have even been facing surgery.

I recommend that anyone who is experiencing any type of pain come here. It certainly worked for me!

— **Robert M.**

· · · · ·

46
Herniated Discs

Dr. Paul Baker has enabled me to walk again without pain and without limping.

I developed severe pain with sciatica in my right leg at age 56. The MRI showed 2 herniated discs. Being a nurse anesthetist, many of the nurses and physicians I worked with who had back problems and opted for surgery, some having 2 or 3 back surgeries, resulted in continued back problems. Therefore, I decided back surgery was not for me. I would just live with the pain.

At age 60, I joined BEAT Training and my trainer recommended Dr. Paul. I was very skeptical, but I decided to see if chiropractic treatment would help relieve my sciatic pain. I was completely amazed when my sciatic pain was cured.

Then I made a big mistake, I stopped going to therapy once the pain was gone. At age 64, I developed arthritis in my right knee with severe leg pain. My x-rays showed both meniscus torn so I had arthroscopy but continued with leg pain and limping. After suffering for another year, I came back to Dr. Paul Baker. Again, with chiropractic treatment, my leg pain and limp were cured.

I have learned that chiropractic care is necessary for one's neuromuscular well-being. I will never again stop receiving chiropractic care and I want to thank Dr. Paul for returning me to a normal and active lifestyle.

— Jessica S.

• • • • •

Dr. G, I wanted to take a few minutes to write you a quick note on my progress but before I do I should tell you how all my back pain started.

On 6-5-15 Amy (my fiance) and I took a trip out of town to Gatlinburg. Early Saturday morning, I woke up to use the bathroom and jumped out of bed to the most horrific pain I've ever felt before. At the time I didn't know what it was. I managed to lay down on the floor, thinking that if I could just stretch it out, everything would be okay. That was further from the truth because the more I tried to stretch the worse the pain got.

On plan for this trip was to go horseback riding, hiking and ziplining but because the pain only got worse we were not able to do any of those things. Amy and I walked to the nearest drugstore to get pain medication. I bought two bottles of back pain pills and immediately took 3-4 pills and then another 3-4 pills and then another set of pills. By noon I had consumed over 15 pills. The pain did go down but my left leg started to get numb, which concerned me greatly because I've never had that feeling before. I tried to find a doctor but none were available on a Saturday in a small town.

The next day I took another 15 plus pills to control the pain but on Monday when I woke up the pain got even worse. I took 15 pills again but I think I became immune to them because they didn't help. I called work to get the day off and got the earliest appointment to see a doctor. In less than 4 minutes from the start of my visit, I'm out of the doctor's office with stronger prescription medications. He couldn't tell me what was wrong until I got an MRI. He just wrote me a prescription. The next day I got the MRI and the day after that I went back to the doctor to see the results.

A herniated disk is what I had. I didn't know what it was or what it meant. The doctor quickly suggested I go see a surgeon to see if I needed surgery. I didn't know what to think. I was mad and afraid at the same time. I started to research online for natural ways to fix my herniated disc. I found YouTube videos titled "how to treat your own back" using the McKenzie method. I watched every video on it and did the exercises. Finally I was at least able to walk but the pain was definitely still present because I couldn't stand up straight and I couldn't stand for more than 2 minutes straight but I could at least walk and sit down.

At this point, I had hope that I could get better without surgery but I knew it was going to be a long process. I was very sad and even depressed for a while. Prior to my injury I was very active, working out 6 times a week and some days even twice a day. I love the gym and working out. As I laid on the floor for many hours I wondered if I would ever get back to the gym. This was a very sad moment in my life.

The surgeon's office kept calling me to set up an appointment but I kept ignoring them. Finally I answered and told them I would not see them because surgery is not an option for me.

I kept watching the YouTube videos and doing the back exercises determined that I was going to get better on my own. One of the videos I was about to watch had an ad popup with the Baker brothers, the ad kept me watching because a lady was telling her story on how Baker Chiropractic and Wellness helped her prevent a 3rd surgery and how her pain level went from a 9-10 on a daily basis down to a 1.

I immediately took the number down and called your office first thing the next morning. The lady who answered the phone was so nice and caring. She asked about my situation, she asked if I had heard of the McKenzie method? I'm like "YEA" super excited because at that moment, I knew I was calling the right place. I quickly set up an appointment that same day and that's when I met you Dr. G.

As you already know, I was in very bad shape but fast forward today, six months later...

I can walk normal again

I can run (ran a 5K in September)

I can stand on my calves (I couldn't even do a calf raise on my

left foot with only my body weight)

On a scale of 1-10, the pain is less than a 1, sometimes weeks go by without any pain at all

I'm back to work doing all my normal duties

I can bend down without any pain

I can lift heavy boxes

More importantly I'm back to doing what I love, working out

I'm so thankful that I've met you and the Baker Chiropractic and Wellness family. Because of you I'm now smarter on how to treat my body. I'm getting stronger every time I come visit you but what I'm most excited about is the hope you gave me when I was at my lowest point. Less than 6 months ago I was hopeless on the ground and you've given me my strength back and for that I'm forever grateful.

Thank you for all you have done for me!

Sincerely,

— **Mago M.**

· · · · ·

I've wanted to write my testimony since coming to Dr. Patrick Baker. I just didn't know where to start, so I'll start at the beginning. Over 35 years ago I injured my lower back at home. I went to a chiropractor (not to

this one) for a brief time with no relief. Then I started working at an orthopedic office where I have been for 21 years. One of the doctors there over the years has sent me for epidural injections, nerve blocks, physical therapy, etc. only getting temporary relief ach time. The only thing that I stayed away from was pain medications and I am grateful for that. The last few years I have been getting worse, and even walking crooked. Every step was painful. I also had herniated 2 discs in my neck in 2005.

Sometimes the pain would be so bad, I felt suicidal. I hadn't slept all night long in years. My husband started going to Dr. Baker when he herniated his low back. Shortly after, I had sciatica and Dr. Baker's office got me in that day. I could barely walk in, but only 1 hour later I walked out straight...and straighter than I had been in a long time! I knew right then I had found some hope! I was even able to fly to California to visit my sister. Before then, even a short car ride was painful. Every day is better. I'm even looking forward to resuming my hobbies, which are landscape photography and working in my yard. I would urge anyone who is in pain to not give up and come in to see Dr. Baker. He and his staff are wonderful! It is certainly worth it. Mere words are not enough. And did I forget to mention, I've been going there less than 2 months! It truly will be a Merry Christmas!!

— **Carol R.**

· · · · ·

My name is Ken Rice. I am a 62 yr old man that had never had chiropractic care.

In 2009, I had a total hip replacement which was the result of osteoarthritis. At this time I was given a prescription of Meloxican for the arthritis. Six months later I started having pain in my neck. I went to my primary care and he referred me to a spine surgeon. I was sent for a cat scan with dye. The results came back that I would need to have a procedure to put cadaver bones in my neck due to the osteoarthritis.

After praying about my situation I decided to hold off on the surgery, at which time they recommended I stay on the Meloxican. I was also on blood pressure medications and had been for quite some time.

I am a local beekeeper in Fairfield, Ohio. In the summer of 2012 it was time to extract honey. I was out on one of the farms pulling boxes off the hives that were full of honey. Each box weighs approx. 65-70 lbs. I must have turned the wrong way and a pain shot across my lower back and down my left leg. I thought I strained something and with some rest, it would be ok. The pain didn't go away. So I went to my primary care physician. They took x-rays and sent me to a neurosurgeon. He said I had a herniated disc and we would try epidural injections. I went thru a series of those with little or no results. All the time remaining in almost unbearable pain. I couldn't stand walk or lie down without the pain. I was desperate for some relief and I didn't know where to turn.

A wonderful friend that goes to our church (Geneva Lewis) begged me to go see Dr. Patrick Baker. This was approximately 2 months after I had injured my back. The day of the appointment I could barely walk into the office. I was slumped over and the pain was obvious on my face. Dr. Baker's staff greeted me and took me right back and did x-rays and scanned my back. The scan showed my neck and left lower back were severe. I waited in the doctor's and the Dr. walked in and said, "Mr. Rice, we are going to help you."

They had me hang over a machine as long as I could. He adjusted me and when I got up off that table I was standing straight and my pain was decreased by 40%. I could not believe what one visit did for my pain. With every visit to Dr. Patrick Baker's office, my back continued to improve until I was pain free!

We are still working on my neck, which was more severe than my back. I have so much confidence in Dr. Baker and his amazing staff, that I know we will get my neck pain free also.

My wife Carol and I took a 30 day challenge that the Baker Chiropractic clinic offered. It was literally a life changing experience for us. We were to use recipes from the Maximized Living nutritional plans, a book offered at Dr. Patrick Baker's office. We weighed in on a machine that told your weight, body fat percentage, and muscle mass. After the weigh in, we started our 30 day challenge. The recipes in the book I will have to say are absolutely delicious. We started every morning with a protein shake which was a scoop of Maximized Living Protein powder. That is added to 1 cup of almond milk. To that I would add fresh Kale, fresh strawberries, fresh pineapple, a few almonds. The book is a wealth of knowledge for nutritional values on various things. For example, you would need to eat 20 bowls of oatmeal to equal the nutritional value of 1 bowl of Kale. I put the fresh kale in the protein shake and when you blend it up you don't even taste the kale. After a couple weeks we realized this was a life style change we could live with. We both work, so what makes it nice is any of the recipes can be done in 20 minutes or less. The recipes literally explode with flavor. After 30 days we weighed in. I lost 14.2 lbs. and reduced my body fat by 2.8%. My wife did even better reducing her body fat by 3.6%.

An added amazing fact is that both my wife and I are off all prescription medications including blood pressure, arthritis meds, acid reflux meds and cholesterol meds. Just as a side note. The acid reflux was caused by the extended use of the arthritis med.

It is now 6 1/2 weeks and I am down 20 lbs. and my wife Carol is doing as well. We monitor our blood pressure every morning just to keep tabs. So far both are at or slightly below normal with no medications. We are at a point in our lives that we are living a much healthier life because of the total program Dr. Patrick Baker and his amazing staff offer for everyone. It's not a diet. It's keeping your spine in alignment and discovering a nutritional plan you can follow and enjoy for the rest of your life.

I thank God for directing our path to Dr. Patrick Baker and his staff. Dr. Baker and his staff truly care about your quality of life. My wife and I are living proof.

— **Ken R.**

· · · · ·

47
Hiatal Hernia

One night I went to bed and woke up with terrible chest sensations and a handful of other symptoms. At the time, I was almost certain that it was a heart attack.

I was brought to the E.R. where the doctors did a hand full of tests on me. I had blood work done, multiple EKG's, chest x rays and even a CT scan. All the tests came back perfect. I finally had an endoscopy done and that's when I was diagnosed with a hiatal hernia.

At this point I was happy that they finally found out what was wrong with me, until I found out that there seemed to be virtually no reliable way to repair the problem.

I had heard horror stories about the surgery so I concluded that I would never consider it.

Being the investigative person that I am, I started to look on the web for other options. And one day I was blessed enough to come across Baker Chiropractic's website. I read a few testimonials and was eager to try the chiropractic route. I had never been to a chiropractor before so I was a bit nervous. But I can assure you it was one of the best decisions I have ever made in my entire life.

After my very first hiatal hernia chiropractic adjustment I felt relief and was eating more the next day. Now, after just a week and a half of treatment I feel like the hiatal hernia is completely going away.

Baker Chiropractic and Wellness is fantastic and I can assure you, if you are coming from out of state it is 100% worth the trip!

— **Liam K.**

. . . . .

I was diagnosed with a hiatal hernia 15 years ago. I took Nexium for frequent heartburn.

The day I pushed open and walked through Dr. Baker's office door was a big turning point for me and my health issues.

I am impressed with the precise manipulations of my diaphragm along with the constant encouragement and support given to me by Dr. Paul Baker and Dr. Todd Worthington.

Most of all, I am impressed with the surprising results!

My positive results didn't happen immediately. It took my perseverance and my trust in both Dr. Paul and Dr. Todd. These were the keys to feeling better and ending years of expensive and damaging medications.

I encourage anybody to at least try Baker Chiropractic and Wellness and their approach for hiatal hernias.

The results will amaze you!

— **Eliane Y.**

· · · · ·

I started care with Dr. Joe Fields at Baker Chiropractic and Wellness five months ago in search of relief from persistent hiatal hernia discomfort.

I had never been to a chiropractor before but was willing to try in order to avoid surgery and taking medications on a long-term basis.

A few weeks into treatment I started noticing improvement and could go about my daily routine without my symptoms being aggravated. In addition to this, Dr. Joe has gladly worked to improve my spinal curvature and the tightness in my jaw and wrists. I never expected to have all of these issues addressed at a chiropractor, much less in such an effective manner.

I would recommend others see Dr. Joe Fields for his compassionate and skilled approach in addressing a wide array of health concerns.

I thank the team at Baker Chiropractic and Wellness for providing me with excellent care and a renewed sense of optimism regarding the state of my health.

— **Rachel L.**

• • • • •

For over 10 years, I have struggled off and on with digestive issues. My symptoms have included upset stomach, cramping, acid reflux, bile reflux, and stomach gastritis.

I have been through just about every test traditional doctors can give including 2 upper digestive tract scopes, gallbladder ultrasound, gallbladder dye test, ct scan, and MRI.

Through all this testing, it was decided that removing my gallbladder was the best option and boy this was not the case as it only made things worse as I continued to struggle with my digestion.

Through the years since my surgery and through a lot of self education I have cleaned up my diet removing inflammatory foods like gluten and dairy. I was feeling better until last year when my symptoms returned again. I began getting extreme acid reflux as soon as I would start eating and after it happened twice in one week I knew I had to do something.

So I pulled out the paperwork from one of my scope tests done years ago and noticed that I had a hiatal hernia. Not wanting to go down the same testing path as I have already done, I got on the internet and Googled hiatal hernia treatment and to my relief I found Dr. Baker's website. So I set up a consultation and met Dr. Baker and went through the first treatment and I immediately felt better. We finished the treatment protocol and my symptoms have vanished.

Dr. Baker explained to me that the actual cause of the problem were subluxations in my spine which were blocking the nerve flow to these organs. I couldn't be more impressed with Dr. Baker; this guy really understands how the body works and goes out of way to help you get better. I would also like to say the friendly atmosphere in the office is also top notch as his staff are just as dedicated as he is in helping his patients get better and really care about each patient.

My only regret is I wish I would have discovered this treatment option sooner. Thanks again Dr. Baker and his staff for helping me tackle this decade long medical problem in such a short time period.

I look forward to coming back for regular check ups to keep my health in top shape.

– Rod M.

· · · · ·

I came to Baker Chiropractic after being coerced by my daughter. I was quite skeptical and only going for her. But, at 82 years old I was told by my regular doctor that surgery was too dangerous for me for one, because of my age and two, because I have two leaky heart valves.

Not wanting to give up, she found others mention relief with Chiropractic care. My diagnosis was a large hiatal hernia. This was first discovered 40+ years ago, however, most recently my stomach had moved all the way up past my diaphragm and was pressing against one of my lungs causing it to be caved in at least 50%. This made it very hard to do much of anything anymore. I struggled with shortness of breath, walking and just living everyday life as I was accustom to. Eating resulted in immediate discomfort with gas, belching and indigestion. I was unable to do anything for at least ½ hour after eating.

My doctor said my hernia was the largest hiatal hernia he had ever seen. 3-4 years ago I was able to walk 8 miles almost daily. Now, I was unable to walk a block or go up one flight of stairs without being completely out of breath.

After approximately 3 treatments at Baker Chiropractic I could notice a substantial improvement and decided to continue therapy. My daughter said she noticed the very next time we ate together. I am not completely cured and due to age and the severity of the hernia, I still have symptoms. However, they are greatly improved and I am able to better function in life and have more comfort. I can breathe easier and eating is not near as miserable and something that stops me in my tracks.

Though not walking miles as I used to, I am able to walk much more comfortably and not have as much difficulty in my breathing. Thank you Baker Chiropractic!

— **John W.**

• • • • •

After having significant pain in my abdomen due to a hiatal hernia for many months, and not receiving a clear treatment plan from traditional medical protocol, I called Dr. Paul Baker to see if he could help.

Dr Paul told me that he could treat and completely fix the hernia through adjusting my stomach out of my esophagus and that my wounded abdomen would heal on its own.

This was a simple but surprising solution since many of my friends thought that surgery was the only solution for any kind of hernia.

I am now about finished with my treatment and feel completely healed, back to normal, and pain-free. Thanks so much!

— **Ethan S.**

· · · · ·

It started on February 16th when I went to a local area medical clinic with symptoms of extreme fatigue, fever and coughing. I was examined, swabbed and diagnosed with Type B Flu.

The following Sunday, I was experiencing severe chest pains and pressure. I was taken to the ER where they took two chest x-rays, an EKG and did blood work. They diagnosed me with Pleurisy which is inflammation of the tissues that line the lungs and chest cavity. I was told the Pleurisy was a result of my coughing from the Flu.

Nearly three weeks later on March 13th, I went to Urgent Care with severe chest pains, pressure and shortness of breath. I had two more chest x-rays taken, another EKG and more blood work. I was then sent back to the hospital for a CT scan with a dye to check for blood clots in my lungs. After all of these tests, x-rays and scans, the diagnosis was once again Pleurisy from the coughing associated with the Flu even though the coughing had stopped.

A week later, the same symptoms I had been experiencing were getting worse. It felt at times as if I were having a heart attack. The ER doctor sent me to a cardiologist where I had a stress test on a treadmill and an ultrasound of my heart. Nothing was found and again I was diagnosed with Pleurisy.

After dealing with all this for well over a month, I was desperate to find out why I kept having shortness of breath, pain, and tightness in my chest. It almost felt like a balloon was being blown up in my chest.

I called Dr. Paul Baker at Baker Chiropractic and Wellness on a

Saturday afternoon and left a message that I needed his advice. He called me back Saturday evening very concerned and suggested I meet him on a Sunday at his office for an evaluation. Within five minutes of my visit, Dr. Baker diagnosed a hiatal hernia. He explained how the hiatal hernia was the source of the pressure in my chest. He also described how acid reflux from the hiatal hernia was causing sharp pains.

Dr. Baker confidently assured me he could fix the hernia but warned it would be a bit uncomfortable. With both of his hands, he put pressure under my ribcage and slowly pushed the hernia back down thru my diaphragm. When I stood up, I had instant relief! Both the pain and pressure I had felt for over a month was gone.

After many sleepless nights in fear that I was having a heart attack, after multiple visits to the hospital, urgent care and even a cardiologist, Dr. Baker diagnosed and fixed the pain that I was having in one 20-minute Sunday afternoon visit to his office! He continues to check my hernia when I come in for my regular visits and it seems to be fine.

In thinking back when I had the Flu, I remember coughing so hard at one point that it felt like something ripped in my stomach. I'm now convinced this was the start of the hiatal hernia.

I am both amazed and extremely disappointed that with all of the x-rays, CT scans, blood work and series of other tests over a period of 40+ days, a correct diagnosis could not be made. Equally shocking were my medical bills. The cost of following traditional medical care guidance and instructions exceeded $30,000!!! This doesn't take into account the cost of the mental anguish of not knowing what was wrong with me, thinking I was having a heart attack and the constant worry and stress placed on our entire family.

I am very grateful to Dr. Paul Baker for his incisive diagnosis and his immediate and successful treatment of my hiatal hernia.

— **Terri B.**

· · · · ·

48
High Blood
Pressure

I came to Dr. Baker back in February 2008. I was having neck pain and my blood pressure was elevated. After doing some x-rays, we found out my neck had no curvature, my hips were off by 14 millimeters which is a lot in the
chiropractic field and my back needed some adjusting.

Since then Dr. Baker has been able to eliminate my neck pain and reduce my blood pressure to a normal level. I'm scheduled to have follow-up x-rays in September when I go to a monthly maintenance schedule. I'm sure my neck and spine will be greatly improved thanks to Dr. Baker.

I also want to comment on Dr. Baker's staff. Jennifer, Courtney, and Danielle are some of the nicest people you will ever meet.

They definitely make you feel like you're at home when you're in the office. They are always willing to help you and answer any questions that you may have. I wish more doctors' offices were like Dr. Baker's office.

— **C. Weber**

• • • • •

49
High Cholesterol

My name is Vicki and like many people, I developed high cholesterol. I work in healthcare as a radiological technician and realize how high cholesterol is a major risk factor for things like heart disease and heart attacks.

I talked to my medical doctor about my high cholesterol levels who recommended I start taking a prescription cholesterol medication to manage my cholesterol levels.

Not being a fan of taking medications and dependent on prescription drugs to live my life, I decided to look at other options. After doing some research, I found Baker Chiropractic and Wellness and their all natural cholesterol reduction program. I read stories submitted by their patients who found success with lowering their cholesterol levels with this program, so I decided to schedule an appointment.

After meeting with Dr. Patrick Baker and his wonderful staff, I was convinced Baker Chiropractic's Cholesterol Reduction Program was the right answer for me.

After about three months in their cholesterol reduction program, I decided to return to my medical doctor to have blood work done. When the results came back from the lab, my medical doctor was shocked by how much my cholesterol levels had gone down!

Here are the numbers at the start of my cholesterol reduction program at Baker Chiropractic and the numbers after three months in the program:

Cholesterol Level September 2014 = 261

Cholesterol Level December 2014 = 221 (Lowered my cholesterol by 40 points!)

HDL – Sept. = 62

HDL – Dec. = 66 (HDL is the good cholesterol, increased that by 4 points!)

LDL – Sept. = 171

LDL – Dec. = 134 (LDL is the bad cholesterol, decreased that by 37 points!)

Triglycerides – Sept. = 131

Triglycerides – Dec. = 106 (Lowered triglycerides (fat in blood) by 25 points!)

My experience with Baker Chiropractic and Wellness has done so much more than just lower my cholesterol level. They've taught me about my body, how I can take care of it to prevent disease and how to live a life of health and wellness. It's changed my life and my future.

— Vicki L.

· · · · ·

I have been a patient of Dr. Paul Baker's since June 2010. I started treatment at Dr. Paul's Red Bank facility for low back pain issues. Dr. Baker is a very "holistic" doctor, concerned about the patient's entire health. I had been taking a statin for high cholesterol since

April of 2010, prescribed by my cardiologist. After about 4 months, I started experiencing severe pain in my hip and hand joints. Dr. Baker recommended that I stop taking the statin and try a natural supplement to treat the high cholesterol.

I began a regimen of taking EFAs – Essential Fatty Acids along with Niacin (Vitamin B). My cholesterol was tested at 259 (HDL-45, LDL-175, and Triglycerides-195). After being on the all-natural regimen for 3 months, my cholesterol dropped to 197 (HDL-82, LDL-99, Triglycerides-81). I was amazed at the increase in HDL without adding any exercise. I am expecting even better results once I increase exercise and have been on this all-natural regimen for a longer period of time. Thank you Dr. Baker!

— B. McCormick

50
Hip Pain

I decided to get chiropractic work done because I am on my third pregnancy and had a lot of back pain and hip pain. It was incredibly uncomfortable and my acid reflux was awful.

I've only been here now about 4 visits, and I am feeling absolutely no back pain or hip pain! My acid reflux has diminished quite a bit too and now pains that I didn't even realize were there are diminishing as well!

I'm feeling a lot better, my sleep is no longer disrupted, and my mood towards my family is better. I can move around better, and I am not "waddling" as much. I am walking more.

Thank you Dr. Mike and Baker Chiropractic!

— Mandy T.

Thank you Dr. Kelly (Duffner)! You are such a weekly encouragement to me. I remember the day I limped into your office with extreme right hip pain and Kaleb said, "We're going to help you Merry!"

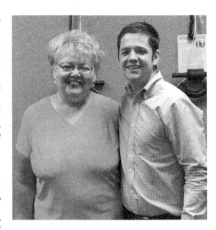

I believe in chiropractic care, but I have to say, I've never experienced the level of care that I have received at Baker Chiropractic and Wellness in any other doctors' offices.

Before coming here, I was prescribed a Prednisone Burst for 5 days. It was not helping so I turned to chiropractic care. I had gone to a chiropractor years ago for my back. Therefore, I wasn't skeptical at all when I came here. I was just hoping and praying that Dr. Kelly could help me.

Four months after coming to Baker Chiropractic and Wellness, the pain has diminished greatly and I'm improving weekly. I can walk again. I am so much better and looking forward to resuming my daily 4.5 mile walks.

It's so nice to have a doctor that truly cares about you. I feel welcomed and loved. It's great to be able to trust someone and know they are going to really help you... not just put a Band-Aid on the problem.

Your office staff is kind and helpful. You really care about me!

If I would have not come here, I would still be in a lot of pain and on medications that only mask the pain instead of getting rid of it.

— Merry T.

• • • • •

I have had extreme low back pain, hip pain and leg pain for well over ten years which greatly limited my normal, day-to-day activities.

In my search for help with my pain issues, I would have done just about anything to get relief!

My many visits to a local chiropractor and physicians proved futile. I endured various scans, tests and procedures only to realize that it was a complete waste of my time and effort. I was getting worse and could not even enjoy being a Dad to my son!

It was then that a co-worker told me about Dr. Patrick Baker at Baker Chiropractic and Wellness.

My first adjustment seemed to be somewhat painful but when I stood up, I quickly realized that my long term pain was GONE! I was, and continue to be AMAZED at my ongoing progress!

No more pain when getting in and out of my vehicle. No more discomfort when sitting or driving for an extended period of time!

Now I can play with my son! My pain is gone! It really is!

Thank you Dr. Baker and staff!

You have all been God's hand extended to me!

— Andrew S.

My name is Marlene and I was at the point of thinking "If this is what growing old is like, it's no fun!"

I had neck pain and back problems for 20+ years. I always felt sick and was unable to look up or turn my head. I couldn't do things I enjoy like gardening or slow dancing. I couldn't hug anyone or turn my head to chat with someone.

I started chiropractic care as a last chance before having to undergo neck surgery. When I started to see signs of recovery with chiropractic care, I knew this was the answer and I wanted total and complete recovery.

Not only did I get mobility back with my neck and back but I found I could now lay on my right side without immediate dizziness.

Recently, my family doctor said I had arthritis in my wrists. Oh my aching hands. Dr. Joe Fields took a look and fixed them with just one adjustment. He takes care of my wrists every week now. No more aching!

After chiropractic care at Baker Chiropractic and Wellness, I can now:

- Look up
- Hug people

- Lay down however I want without dizziness
- Turn my head from side-to-side
- Hold my head up

I also had no idea chiropractic care could fix my aching hands and in the last two weeks, I can breath with my mouth closed. No more snoring!

I got my life back. I can live because I can move!

My name is Tim and I had been struggling with headaches, lower back pain and hip problems for a few years. I was diagnosed with osteoarthritis and given pain killers for the hip pain. I eventually had both hips replaced and I couldn't do much of anything.

The chiropractic care I have received at Baker Chiropractic and Wellness gives me energy, mobility and just makes me feel better overall. I would not be able to work 12+ hour days without chiropractic care. I am also sick far less and haven't had a case of the flu since coming here.

— Marlene and Tim M.

· · · · ·

I reluctantly made an appointment with Baker Chiropractic and Wellness for my 12 year old daughter due to hip pain, back pain and knee pain she had been experiencing for about one year.

Although we had sought chiropractic care elsewhere,

months prior to our first appointment with Dr. Patrick Baker, Brooke's pain continued and actually got worse over time. I had also taken Brooke to see a specialist at Children's Hospital for a pricey exam and x-rays. The doctor at Children's Hospital explained to us that Brooke was suffering from "Growing Pains". Not the case!

The chiropractic treatments she was receiving from previous chiropractors seemed to help for a temporary time, but always resurfaced shortly after her treatments. This is why I was not optimistic about seeking additional chiropractic care for my daughter ... because the treatments previous to Baker Chiropractic and Wellness were not successful or long lasting.

Much to my surprise, we walked into Dr. Patrick's office and after one visit, I was feeling like we were finally in the right place! Not only because Dr. Baker and his ENTIRE staff were warm, friendly, caring, knowledgeable, and accommodating, but because they had such a comprehensive system in place to truly assess the patient's issues and aggressively solve those issues!

I felt comfortable about their plan because they educated us on how chiropractic care works and how they were planning to help us. There was no mystery or uncertainty after they explained their approach and plan. I also felt comfortable asking Dr. Baker and all of the staff members any questions I may have had. The only surprise was how quickly my daughters pain was relieved after only a few visits.

Brooke was examined, x-rayed and weighed on the scale by Dr. Patrick. As it turns out, my daughter weighed 11 pounds more on her left side than her right due to hip placement issues! I was shocked. She also had alignment problems with her spine and neck. I am grateful to say she weighed only 3 pounds more on her right side after only 2 months of treatment! And after about 8 months of treatment she is pain free and fully mobile and flexible!

Before Dr. Patrick treated her, Brooke was complaining daily of pain when she walked through Kings Island, cheered or tumbled. Brooke is now pain free and is walking, cheering and tumbling with great success and pleasure, thanks to Dr. Baker and his wonderful staff!

Baker Chiropractic and Wellness truly cares about their patients. My daughter looks forward to seeing Dr. Patrick for each visit, not only because he alleviated her pain, but also because he is so kind and gentle. He and his staff do whatever it takes to help her and I appreciate their professionalism and attentiveness!

I have total faith and confidence in Dr. Baker and his staff and I am grateful to them for improving my daughter's quality of life!

In short ... they really know what they are doing and they do it well!

Thank you, Dr. Baker and thanks to your competent staff.

— **Betsy T.**

• • • • •

51
Hypothyroidism

About two years ago after my mother had been diagnosed with thyroid cancer so, I had my thyroid levels checked and found out that I had hypothyroidism.

Up to this point I was quite healthy and active and would have never thought there was anything wrong. Because of my mother's history and the fact that my numbers were still high after going on Levothyroxine, I began seeing an endocrinologist. She and I began tracking my numbers which had dropped from the original TSH of 9 down to 3.4. I still didn't have a lot of issues that many people who suffer from hypothyroidism tend to have, such as abnormal weight gain, hair loss, fatigue, and many more.

After seeing my doctor for about a year with appointments every three months and adjusting my medications, more hypothyroid related symptoms began appearing. The first problem was numbness in my hands and legs which my primary care doctor thought could be carpel tunnel. However, the endocrinologist knew the direct link that the thyroid has to the nervous system and she said that was probably the problem and we would keep an eye on it.

As time went on more and more issues with nerves and other systems began appearing, such as irregular menstrual cycles. Again we thought it was a complication of my thyroid which was causing this problem, but I went to my gynecologist to have it checked. I then had to have ultrasounds and other tests done to determine where this new set of issues was coming from which led right back to my thyroid.

It wasn't until about 8 months ago that the final issue struck which was my back. Up until this point I thought my back pain was some symptom of all the other issues that had been taking place and the battle I was having with my thyroid. Then as I was going to pick up a piece of paper off the floor my lower back went out. I could barely walk and standing for long periods of time was difficult to stay the least. After suffering from this back pain for about two weeks I decided I needed to have someone look at it because it wasn't getting better. Not wanting to have medicines and surgery as the only fix I went to see Dr. Paul Baker.

Dr. Paul informed me that my back was quite bad in many different places but that he could definitely help me but it would take some work. I also learned that when you have subluxations of the spine that it affects every part of your body. Dr. Paul and I discussed a treatment plan and how I would probably start to see a lot of my health issues start disappearing or even improve.

After six months I am glad to report that all my thyroid related symptoms are completely better. I no longer have any numbness or shooting pains in my hands or feet. Plus my numbers on my thyroid have now been in the normal range of 1.4 for about five months I couldn't' be happier. I am hoping that with continued help from Dr. Paul that I will be able keep my thyroid levels down and all the symptoms at bay.

— **Shelley S.**

52
Indigestion

I started coming to Baker Chiropractic because I was having a lot of indigestion and pain in my middle back.

In 2 months times, my indigestion is gone and I no longer have middle back pain.

— Justine

53
Infant Care

My son Jackson's birth was very traumatic. He was an emergency forceps delivery. He wasn't breathing upon birth and had to be put on a mechanical ventilator and sent to Cincinnati Children's Hospital NICU. He stayed there for a week where we were informed that an MRI showed some damage to his brain in the frontal lobe. As a result of his birth trauma and/or the damage to his brain, Jackson's arm movements and range of motion were drastically affected. He couldn't lift his arms above his head and he carried his arms in a "bulldog" position.

In trying to address this issue, we were sent first to a physical therapist and then an occupational therapist. Neither could figure out the root of the problem with his arms. The occupational therapist actually referred us to an orthopedic surgeon and suggested that surgery might be a possibility. At that time, Jackson was 5 months old and we were still seeing the same issues with limited range of motion and abnormal posture. I decided it was time to try something else.

I researched a bit and found that the doctors at Baker Chiropractic and Wellness had the best reputation in the area with infants. I made an appointment, not sure what to expect. At our first appointment, Dr. Paul explained that Jackson's issues were probably caused by the trauma to his neck and spine when the forceps were used at birth. We started out with an intensive plan, going to see Dr. Paul three times a week. Dr. Paul was very gentle with Jackson's adjustments – Jack generally smiled and babbled the whole time!

Jack is now 7 months old and has a full range of motion after less than 2 months of Dr. Paul's care. We are very grateful to Dr. Paul and his staff for helping our son. His posture now looks very typical, and every time I see him stretch with his arms above his head, I breathe a sigh of relief!"

— B. Martin

• • • • •

54
Infertility

My husband and I were trying to have a baby for a long time. After months of trying and still no baby, I knew I had to try something else. I decided to start going to the chiropractor. I went in to see Dr. Baker and told him my issue. I started adjustments for one (1) month and the next month I was pregnant!

My baby girl, Ellie, was born March 28, 2013, three weeks early. The first month she was having gas pains and not pooping and spitting up constantly. I took her to the Pediatrician and he said that she could go a full month without pooping, which to anyone doesn't seem logical. He said since she was early that her Sphincter needs to loosen up and that takes time. He said that he was going to put her on medicine for Acid Reflux, which I said no, as Ellie was only one month old. I immediately took her to Dr.

Patrick Baker and told him the issue and he immediately said he could help with a smile on his face.

He adjusted her neck and back on a Monday afternoon. From Monday to Wednesday (the next time we saw him) she had pooped eight times and her spitting up had decreased which means Happy Mommy and Daddy.

For the first few months of her life, she saw Dr. Patrick Baker almost three times a week. Now, she goes every few weeks and is the happiest baby. I get compliments all the time for her being so happy and I always say it's because of chiropractic care. She has been sleeping through the night since she has been six weeks old, again, because of her adjustments.

A month ago, Ellie had a temperature for a few days and nothing I done would relieve it. She wouldn't sleep or eat. The Pediatrician said that she had a virus and really couldn't help. I called and talked to Dr. Brock and he came in on a Sunday to adjust her. Her fever was gone by that evening and we all got some sleep. I can't thank him enough for taking the time to come in on a weekend to help my little girl.

In closing, when we go to the office, Ellie immediately hears Dr. Patrick's or Dr. Brock's voice and smiles and giggles. She loves it there.

I just want to thank Dr. Patrick Baker, Dr. Brock, their staff and their families for the help and relief they have given my family.

— **Megan N.**

· · · · ·

55
Insomnia

"Before going to seek treatment from Dr. Garrett Knuckles at Baker Chiropractic and Wellness, I was experiencing neck pain, lower back pain, sharp pain in my left arm and I was walking with a limp. I was also experiencing numbness in my hips which was keeping me up at night.

Dr. Garrett started me on a regiment of adjustments and in as little as four months I am now able to sleep through the night, I am practically pain free, and my limp no longer exists!

My life is so much better now thanks to Dr. Garrett and his staff!"

— **Norma S.**

• • • • •

I suffered from insomnia for over 15 years. I remember the

first episode when I was 12 years old like it was yesterday.

I had a pretty traumatic childhood and learned to essentially sleep with one eye open every night. It was always very limiting on my daily activities, even as a child. I always felt very tired and worn down. I never had any energy or desire to do anything and this continued into my adult life. I had to force myself to get out of bed every day due to sheer exhaustion. Any little sound or movement would wake me up at night and it sometimes took me several hours to be able to fall back to sleep.

At about age 18, I started taking over the counter sleep aids. I tried multiple brands for several months, and after awhile each one would stop working because my body adjusted to it so quickly since I needed to take them every night before bed. I eventually went to my primary doctor and later to a neurologist where I was prescribed sleeping pills for many years. We would try one and when it would stop working, I would be given a prescription for something else. This cycle went on for over 10 years. All the pills they put me on would make me feel groggy and tired the next day and it was supposed to help me feel less like that. I felt like I was in a foggy, dazed state. I began to run on auto-pilot and never had a feeling of true "rest", no matter how much sleep I would get.

I was missing a lot of work due to my lack of sleep. I wasn't able to spend any quality time with my friends or family. My husband grew very frustrated because I was frequently complaining of being tired and exhausted, and yet I was sleeping more and more. It didn't make any sense to him why I was so tired every day, and I couldn't explain it. I never had any energy or desire to do anything, no matter how much sleep the pills gave me. I had not interest in doing anything but laying around and trying to nap. We started to grow apart right under my nose, and I wasn't aware it was happening until much later.

I had been having some sever pain in my neck and left shoulder for many years, and that's what prompted my search for a chiropractor. I looked online and found Baker Chiropractic. They were less than a mile from where I worked at the time. When I called the office, I was able to get in that same evening and had my consultation and exam with Dr. Paul Baker. I got to the office and I couldn't believe how different everything was from all the multiple other doctor's offices I had been to over the years. They all actually cared about what I was going through. They didn't want me to be reliant on medication anymore. I remember leaving the office that first night telling myself not to get too excited because I had no prior success.

After making the decision that I didn't want to keep taking pills anymore, I slowly weaned off my heavy dose of prescription sleeping medications with the help of Dr. Paul. Over time, I was able to fall asleep on my own! That was something that I hadn't been able to do for so many years. It took about 4-5 months to have a good night's sleep with absolutely no pills whatsoever. I never gave up, even though there were some nights that I only slept for an hour or two. I now sleep without the aid of any sleeping medications, natural or prescription, and I am able to sleep through the entire night! I am getting deep, restful, and productive sleep. Something that I thought would never be possible. I am able to function and have so much energy and drive throughout the day, even when I have to get up before the sun comes up!

Before becoming a patient of Baker Chiropractic and Wellness, I was all around miserable. I had so many health problems, most

56
Intercostal
Neuralgia

Intercostal neuralgia is a health condition that causes pain with the intercostal nerves. These nerves are located between your ribs. Margaret came to us with pain in her upper ribs that would travel across her chest. She went to other doctors looking for answers but didn't find them. A friend told her about Dr. Patrick Baker and she

came to us. Dr. Baker diagnosed her pain as chronic intercostals neuralgia. Now, she is pain-free.

"The last part of February 2011 I began to have pain in my left upper ribs. The pain would travel across my chest. I thought I was having a heart attack.

By Dr. Paul Baker, Dr. Patrick Baker and Hundreds of Patients

I went to my primary care doctor and she said it must be from my back and sent me to a pain management clinic. This was after three x-rays, a fully body scan and one shot for pain.

After the first injection, the pain worsened and I was sent for an MRI with contrast. The doctors told me if I was not better after the third injection then I should see another doctor. So, I called my husband's doctor that did his back surgery. After another MRI, he said there was nothing wrong with my back.

After a few months of pain that was getting worse every day, a friend told me about coming to Dr. Patrick Baker. I called and was in the office in just days. When I told Dr. Baker the pain was in my ribs – not my back, he and his staff began treatment that now has me pain-free!

Thank you Dr. Baker and Staff."

— **Margaret K.**

. . . . .

57
Interstitial
Cystitis

My name is Twanna and I have Interstitial Cystitis.

Most of you have probably never heard of it. If you have, you probably have I.C., and wish you hadn't. It is a disease of the bladder where the lining is very thin so your urine is toxic to your bladder. You have the urge to urinate constantly

along with great pain. Currently, the medical field has no known cause and therefore no known cure for interstitial cystitis.

I, like everyone else who has been diagnosed with this disease, went through all the approved "torture". I was at the Emergency Room numerous times and was even told by one of the E.R. nurses to pray for death. There was nothing anyone could do for me. I went through cat scans, M.R. I. scans, biopsies, colonoscopies, stomach scopes, and even laparoscopic surgery before I was diagnosed. All this time my pain scale was at 10 always and I grew more depressed every day. The only answer they gave me was bigger and bigger pain pills. At that point and time, I was happy to get them because the pain was always so great.

Then the fun really began and I was sent to an urologist. Don't get me wrong, they were kind to me and did everything they knew how to do. I started having bladder "cocktails". This was a catheter into my bladder 3 times a week for over a year. I was also put on the drug Elmiron. I don't have to describe how the catheters were, if you have ever had one you know. The Elmiron was very expensive even with good insurance. Its side effects were permanent hair loss and damage to your liver (which you had to check every six months). This process helped some but never got my pain below a 6. Everyday life was a struggle. Keeping positive was a struggle.

Then one day on the internet I typed in the search bar "Hope for Interstitial Cystitis" and Baker Chiropractic and Wellness came up. I read the whole thing on I.C. and how they have helped many people over the years. Was I skeptical? Yes. Was my family skeptical? Yes. But I wanted to try something other than drugs or the dreaded catheter. What did I have to lose?

So I made an appointment and went in and talked to them. I remember crying through the whole first appointment. They seemed so positive that they would be able to help me even though for three years I was told no one could.

So I started going to them three times a week. Getting adjustments and therapy. Gradually my pain started to decrease. Dr. Baker also had me adjust my diet and put me on anti-inflammatory supplements, both of which have also helped greatly. Now my pain stays between a 1 and 2, which to me is a 90% improvement.

I have my life back! I can work and take vacations. Some days it's like I don't have I.C. at all. If I do have a big flare (which doesn't happen as often as it used to), Dr. Baker is great to get me right in and it usually only takes a small amount of time to get the flare back down. Currently, I still see Dr. Baker twice a week and my goal is to be pain free like his other I.C. patients soon.

I am very thankful to have found Dr. Baker at Baker Chiropractic and Wellness and to have been given a chance for a pain free life without all the drugs and medical procedures.

I also want to thank and commend his staff. They are friendly, sympathetic, kind and knowledgeable and do Dr. Baker's office proud. I also want to say that I listen to the comments between Dr. Baker and his other patients. I hear how much he really cares for them and the gratitude and respect they have for him. All of which is rare in today's world in the medical field. Usually you are just another number.

If you have interstitial cystitis and you have tried everything and nothing is working, or you are tired of taking drugs, give Dr. Baker the chance to help you. You have nothing to lose.

Thanks again to Dr. Baker and his staff. May God bless each and every one of you."

— **Twanna A.**

· · · · ·

Update to Twanna's Story

I wanted to provide an update on my experience with Baker Chiropractic and Wellness as of May 2014. It has now been a little over a year since I became a patient.

I had IC for three years before I met Dr. Baker. Prior to coming to Baker Chiropractic, I was in constant pain and having to endure many painful tests. I was also taking strong medications with serious side effects to get a minimum amount of relief.

A little over a year ago I started getting my adjustments and therapy at Baker Chiropractic and Wellness. I started to see a gradual decrease in pain. Doc has stuck with me thru both the good and the bad days. Now I am pain free most days! If I have any pain at all, it is very little.

I thank God every day for Dr. Baker and his staff. I can work again. I can go on vacation. I have my life back.

If you have IC please give them a try!

— **Twanna A.**

· · · · ·

I was battling Interstitial Cystitis or IC for 3 years before meeting Dr. Paul Baker. When my problem first started, I was on antibiotics a number of times which I believe made my situation worse. I was finally diagnosed with IC and prescribed IC medicine. I tried other procedures too like instillation and dilation every 1 or 2 months for more than a year.

Initially, I could control my symptoms to an extent while on medications but as time passed, nothing helped. I grew very tired of regular visits to the doctor's office and spending lots of money. Finally, I decided to restrict my diet and started regular workouts in order to keep my problem minimized. I had become hopeless about a complete cure for my disease.

One Monday morning, I woke up with a severe IC flare-up and my back was hurting too. I thought I had just pulled a muscle from the work I had done over the weekend and my backache would go away. But I wasn't sure what was aggravating my IC pain. I missed work and school for 4 days and tried everything I could think of at home to alleviate my symptoms. On Thursday morning, I was searching the internet for a doctor in Cincinnati that could treat IC and came across the Baker Chiropractic website.

Although I had my doubts about chiropractic care, I wanted to give it a try. I was already hopeless from failed medical treatments for my IC and on top of it, my back was hurting too. After an X-ray, Dr. Paul told me that I had a subluxation for a very long time and all my symptoms were related. Surprisingly, I actually got some relief after my very first chiropractic adjustment which convinced me to continue adjustments. Dr. Paul also suggested a natural detox solution for everyday use which has become my favorite remedy. Now, I can eat and drink regularly.

Within 2-3 weeks, I was completely symptoms free! It's been 2 months and I don't have any IC troubles anymore. I am still getting adjusted in order to completely correct my spine and keep it healthy. I love the many benefits, some which I didn't even expect. I have a healthier abdomen and my chronic dry eye problem is getting better too.

Thanks to Dr. Paul Baker, I would recommend anyone suffering from Interstitial Cystitis to give Baker Chiropractic a try. I believe they will create wonders for you just like they did for me!

— **Divya**

• • • • •

I have been coming to Baker Chiropractic for a variety of medical problems. I am writing to you and asking you to share with everyone a very embarrassing, debilitating and life changing disease that I was diagnosed with in December, 2009.

You have helped me with so many things that I never even thought to ask you if you and chiropractic adjustments could help me with this disease. In October, 2010, when I truly felt at my lowest as my body was filled with pain, I asked you if you could help me with all the excruciating pain I was having. I was diagnosed with Interstitial Cystitis (IC) after going to two of my doctors and having some uncomfortable testing from both doctors. I remember specifically that I asked you in a "whisper", if you could help me with the IC. I didn't want anyone to hear me asking you because it is very difficult to talk about. I couldn't believe it when you told me you had helped other patients with Interstitial Cystitis and you explained how you do this.

As you know, Interstitial Cystitis can be found in both males and females. In my understanding, the inner lining of the bladder becomes inflamed like it is raw inside. This is a problem with all the different kinds of foods and drinks someone consumes. There is a very strict diet for IC and while on this diet, I felt like I was starving and I was still having painful problems. My doctors told me they had no idea what truly causes it. There is only one medicine available at $365.00 per month, taken three times a day and the minor in-office procedures to help with the pain are expensive as well. The IC is extremely painful and can make you urinate up to 60 times a day and the hardest part is the very painful bladder spasms. This is worse than pregnancy or kidney stones.

Dr. Paul, after two adjustments and your manipulations to the correct area of my spine and the nerves to my bladder...the Interstitial Cystitis and all the pain has stopped!! You still give me adjustments in this area on my regular visits and I can't believe I have my life back again...thanks to you!! I had gotten to the point where I didn't leave my home for weeks at a time and you gave me back my freedom. I have no symptoms at all. The pain and spasms are gone. I can't thank you enough for your help these past four years and especially with the IC. I truly hope your patients that may have this disease can come forward to you and let you heal them as you did for me.

With heartfelt thanks...you are definitely my hero and the best Doctor in the USA!'

— Judy

· · · · ·

58
Irritable Bowel Syndrome

"At the age of 19, I was diagnosed with Irritable Bowel Syndrome. Being in horrendous pain and discomfort became normal to me.

I am now 26 and throughout the past 7 years, I have seen several doctors and was prescribed 6 different medications.

The only medication that worked was $207 a month with insurance. It made me feel very nauseated and short of breath.

After seeing Dr Paul Baker for 3 chiropractic adjustments, I saw immediate results. I was able to stop taking the medication and canceled the costly appointments with the specialists.

I would also like to add that everyone at the office is incredibly friendly and welcoming!"

— **Lora S.**

· · · · ·

My name is Marcia Wray. Throughout the 1990's I was seeking treatment for irritable bowel syndrome (IBS). I began with my family doctor, and eventually I sought the services of several specialists, with no results. Every one of these doctors told me that my symptoms were either all in my head, or stress related. I was even told that I should change my career path because there was nothing they could do for me.

In late 1999, while in nursing school, I saw a commercial for Baker Chiropractic recommending chiropractic care for the treatment of IBS. By this time, I was desperate and was willing to try anything. I was quite skeptical of chiropractic doctors because the curriculum in nursing school doesn't speak highly of this type of treatment. But with an open mind I made an appointment to see Dr. Paul Baker in the Redbank office.

Within one week I was seeing substantial results. I was feeling better, I was sleeping better, and I was more comfortable. I didn't have to try out various medications worrying about side effects or go through any embarrassing procedures.

I finished the treatment plan that Dr. Baker set up for me, and was beginning the maintenance plan when I was involved in a car accident in January of 2001. I immediately called Dr. Baker after my accident, and he treated me for neck and back injuries, allowing me to regain full function and continue nursing school.

Once I graduated nursing school, I got married and started a family. Dr. Baker treated me for sciatic pain while I was pregnant, which gave me the ability to walk and sit comfortable during my last trimester. I have since moved to the Fairfield area and I have been working at Bethesda North Hospital for nearly 7 years. And I still see Dr. Patrick Baker, who has treated me for vertigo as well as the aches and pains from working 12 hour shifts as a floor nurse.

No longer skeptical of what chiropractic care can do, I trust both Drs. Baker so much that I have had both of my children in for adjustments, and I have seen instant results with them as well. Symptoms such as ear aches and (believe it or not) the common cold are treated through spinal adjustments, and the symptoms go away much quicker than treating with over-the-counter medications.

I know that if I ever have any questions or concerns, I can call either Dr. Baker at any time, and get a straight answer to my question. I cannot recommend highly enough either of these doctors, and the services they have provided for me and my family have allowed me to live an active and full life.

In a perfect world, where everything is adapted to be 'ergonomically correct', perhaps these services wouldn't be needed. But The demands of nursing – boosting patients, 12+ hour shifts on the concrete floors, and everything else that the hospital (and the patients) throw at you – can wreak havoc on your body. Thanks to Drs. Patrick and Paul Baker, I have been able to comfortably perform my nursing duties, and I have not sustained any work related injury in the process.

— Marcia W, RN

59
Kidney Stones

My first visit to Baker Chiropractic was on January 26th, 2015. I initially came in for injuries from a motorcycle crash in early December 2014 and the subsequent surgery. I started to come in for my back and therapy for my clavicle and neck and the surrounding area. I had been getting adjustments and therapy for a few months and then I also started to have kidney stone problems.

It was after a visit to the emergency room that I found out I was experiencing kidney stones. They sent me home from the ER and told me to come back if things got worse or if I had a fever over 101. I went home exhausted and went to sleep and then only a few hours later I woke up sweating. I took my temperature and it was well over 101. So I immediately went back. They were telling me that I needed to have surgery to get it out.

I was finally back to racing and my normal life at that point and I couldn't imagine having to take even more time out of racing. I talked to Dr. Patrick Baker while I was in the emergency room and decided to not have the surgery. They came in to get me prepped and I told them I was going home.

Dr. Patrick gave me specific "kidney adjustments" and a supplement that helped dissolve the stones so that they could pass. I was scheduled for an Urologist appointment a few days later and they were pressuring me to have the surgery. I started to get mad because they were trying to make me do something that I did not want. I specifically remember telling them "if it makes you feel better then schedule me for the surgery, but I will not show up."

I trusted Dr. Patrick to help get me through the kidney stones just as he helped me heal through my crash injuries and he did. It's impossible to know where I would be without the chiropractic care I have received at Baker Chiropractic and Wellness, but I am very glad that I started going when I did.

Having Dr. Patrick help me with my kidney stones saved me from having to go through more surgeries. They took way longer to pass than I would have liked (if I had the option I would have never had them in the first place!), but they passed and I didn't have to go through any extra misery that the other doctors were trying to do to me.

I am extremely grateful to everyone here for helping me through such tough times.

— Jessica J.

• • • • •

I would like to thank you, Dr. Patrick Baker, for helping with not only with my ongoing back pain but for also offering a solution to my ten week battle with kidney stones.

I first sought out Dr. Baker's help because I threw out my back and could barely move. I was desperate to find relief from my pain as our family had tickets for the All-Star Game festivities. I needed to be on my feet and mobile for the entire week. The treatment I received for my back and shoulder offered relief faster than I expected and I was able to attend all of the events and I could not thank Dr. Baker and his staff enough.

Then at the beginning of September I was rushed to the Emergency Room with severe pain in my left side. The emergency room doctor said I had a 5mm kidney stone and advised me to make an appointment with an urologist but I would have to wait two weeks. The ER supplied me with pain medication and Flow-Max medicines to assist with passing the stone.

The stone did not pass in those two weeks, so the doctor suggested that I give it two more weeks to try to flush it out and if it did not pass by then I would need two rather expensive surgeries.

After the second urologist appointment, I mentioned everything I was going through to Dr. Baker at my very next back therapy session. When we were discussing the options that were presented to me and the cost of the surgeries and Cat Scans. I wasn't sure if he could offer any assistance but he was more than willing to listen when in reality "I was just hoping he could do something to help".

Dr. Baker said there was a kidney stone supplement pill that might be able to help in lieu of the expensive alternatives. I figured what I had nothing to lose, as my trust in Dr. Baker was growing with every visit.

I followed the directions with the supplement taking one week's worth and went back to the doctor and to my surprise they could no longer find the kidney stone on the x-ray. I also had a follow-up visit and they still could not find the kidney stone. I was elated.

So, Dr. Baker saved me from having two surgeries, the cost of the hospital stay, follow up visits and any further doctor visits. The CT scan at the ER alone was $3,186.00, so I can only imagine how much two surgeries would have cost.

I can't thank Dr. Baker and his staff enough for all the help they have given me. My back has felt so much better, I am able to help landscape our yard, tear down our shed and haul away the wood with my children and husband.

Thank you,

— Lori H.

• • • • •

60
Knee Pain

I first stepped foot into Baker Chiropractic because of severe pain radiating in my neck.

I have suffered from recurring whiplash caused from bus accidents as a child that would flare up three to four times a year. I was used to experiencing the pain. But this last flare up wouldn't go away and practically debilitated me.

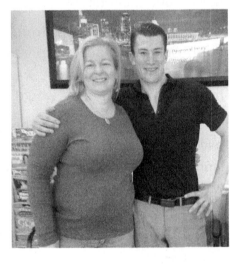

Three weeks later, the stabbing and throbbing pains made it difficult to work, stand, sit, and impossible to drive or sleep. Then I met the great people at Baker Chiropractic and Wellness.

Dr. Brock (Frear) took me under his wing and I saw results within a few visits. He took the time to explain his evaluation of my x rays and to show me the subluxations in my spine that were

By Dr. Paul Baker, Dr. Patrick Baker and Hundreds of Patients

the source of my pain.

In addition to the neck misalignment, Dr. Brock showed me how my hips were also out of alignment. I told him it was probably because I was babying a hurt knee. He replied that my knee was hurting because my hips were offset. He also commented on the fact that he would have thought I had issues with sciatica. My mouth dropped open as I admitted I did have on again/off again sciatic pain.

One adjustment later and I could definitely see a marked difference, not only in my neck but also in my knee. I had more range of motion in my neck, a decrease in pain, I could finally sleep at night, not to mention that I could climb stairs like a normal person again. (side note: I was not at the time suffering from sciatica so I don't know if that was solved or not – but with everything else that improved, I have no doubt that it has as well). After a couple of weeks, I felt like the old me... but better.

It's a joy to go to Baker Chiropractic and Wellness. Not only do I know that I'm correcting my health issues but also the warm and friendly atmosphere is welcoming and makes it a joy to be there. I love the holistic approach and the positivity that radiates the entire practice.

The addition of the massage therapy has helped heal the aches and pains and further preps my muscles and joints to accept the adjustments. And the home therapy gives me the tools to aid me to keep my back healthy.

Dr. Brock and all his staff have a passion for the work they are doing. They each have their own personal story to tell on how chiropractic care, specifically from Baker Chiropractic and Wellness, has enriched their lives and made their health better.

It's refreshing to see people love the work they are doing....to the point where Dr. Brock says this isn't work for him and that he sees it as his joy/mission to help all of us live a happier, healthier life.

I, for one, am greatly appreciative.

I'm a true believer in Chiropractic Care from Baker Chiropractic and Wellness. I came to Baker Chiropractic to alleviate my neck pain but also found the cure for my knee and sciatic pain as well, not to mention making my other internal organs healthier. Life can't get better than that!

— **Patricia B.**

• • • • •

I became a patient of Dr. Baker on August 5, 2011. I could barely walk and I was considering taking a leave of absence from work. The pain was so bad and I had zero energy.

It all started in 2007 when I hurt my knee. My regular physician sent me to physical therapy for my back. I started taking 2-4 Aleve per day. My back felt better but my knee continued to hurt. I began to walk funny because of the knee pain. My whole body got messed up because of my walk.

I was afraid of chiropractic care even though my husband and daughter had been seeing Dr. Baker for over 2 years. I had no choice but to go because by then I had taken more than 2,820

Aleve over the span of 4 years. I bought my Aleve from Sam's Club in the big 500 count bottles and always carried them with me, but now I don't even think about them. I also took Benadryl and Sudafed on a regular basis and ever since my first adjustment I no longer have taken either of those. Also, I had only taken 14 Aleve in the first 2 months of my chiropractic care.

My x-rays showed that I had no curve in my lower back, my spine was crooked and I had a disk pressing into my spinal cord. I'll be honest – the first 4-6 weeks of my care, I felt worse and wanted to quit. Dr. Baker told me to hang in there and that I wasn't going to get better overnight when it took years to get in this shape. By the 10th week, I had energy and was able to move again. Suddenly the pain was disappearing and I was feeling good. I'm not 100% yet, but I am getting there with regular chiropractic adjustments. My whole life is changing because of it.

I'm 58 years old and not ready to sit in a rocker for the rest of my life. I have 8 grandkids with another on the way and a great grandchild due in March. I want to enjoy life with them. I would definitely recommend to everyone to try chiropractic first before giving up or having surgery. Dr. Baker is fantastic and the girls in the office are so sweet and helpful. They make you feel right at home. And if you hurt at anytime, Olivia and Jess will help with therapy.

My knee feels great now! My husband is a Happy Captain and I am his Happy First Mate. Life is worth living again! Thanks Baker Chiropractic!

— **M. Holbert**

. . . . .

I reluctantly made an appointment with Baker Chiropractic and Wellness for my 12 year old daughter due to hip pain, back pain and knee pain she had been experiencing for about one year.

Although we had sought chiropractic care elsewhere, months prior to our first appointment with Dr. Patrick Baker, Brooke's pain continued and actually got worse over time. I had also taken Brooke to see a specialist at Children's Hospital for a pricey exam and x-rays. The doctor at Children's Hospital explained to us that Brooke was suffering from "Growing Pains". Not the case!

The chiropractic treatments she was receiving from previous chiropractors seemed to help for a temporary time, but always resurfaced shortly after her treatments. This is why I was not optimistic about seeking additional chiropractic care for my daughter ... because the treatments previous to Baker Chiropractic and Wellness were not successful or long lasting.

Much to my surprise, we walked into Dr. Patrick's office and after one visit, I was feeling like we were finally in the right place! Not only because Dr. Baker and his ENTIRE staff were warm, friendly, caring, knowledgeable, and accommodating, but because they had such a comprehensive system in place to truly assess the patient's issues and aggressively solve those issues!

I felt comfortable about their plan because they educated us on how chiropractic care works and how they were planning to help us. There was no mystery or uncertainty after they explained their approach and plan. I also felt comfortable asking Dr. Baker and all of the staff members any questions I may have had. The only surprise was how quickly my daughter's pain was relieved after only a few visits.

Brooke was examined, x-rayed and weighed on the scale by Dr. Patrick. As it turns out, my daughter weighed 11 pounds more on her left side than her right due to hip placement issues! I was shocked. She also had alignment problems with her spine and neck. I am grateful to say she weighed only 3 pounds more on her right side after only 2 months of treatment! And after about 8 months of treatment she is pain free and fully mobile and flexible!

Before Dr. Patrick treated her, Brooke was complaining daily of pain when she walked through Kings Island, cheered or tumbled. Brooke is now pain free and is walking, cheering and tumbling with great success and pleasure, thanks to Dr. Baker and his wonderful staff!

Baker Chiropractic and Wellness truly cares about their patients. My daughter looks forward to seeing Dr. Patrick for each visit, not only because he alleviated her pain, but also because he is so kind and gentle. He and his staff do whatever it takes to help her and I appreciate their professionalism and attentiveness!

I have total faith and confidence in Dr. Baker and and his staff and I am grateful to them for improving my daughter's quality of life!

In short ... they really know what they are doing and they do it well!

Thank you, Dr. Baker and thanks to your competent staff.

— **Betsy T.**

· · · · ·

I am a very physically active person. In fact, I am a personal trainer and group fitness instructor. I work-out 6 to 7 days per week. I was experiencing left shoulder pain and left knee pain. I was also getting really congested, had problems breathing and experiencing pain in my lower back. All these problems had been going on for 2-3 years.

Due to the pain, I cut back on my work-out routine. I was limited to what I could do. I wasn't doing much jumping and started doing lighter lifts. I also started adding bands to my work-outs for mobility. I didn't feel like I could give 100%. I cut back on playing pick-up basketball which I love to do. I felt worn down and didn't have much energy because I couldn't give 100%. I was a little depressed because physical activity plays such a big role in my life.

My medical doctor prescribed me an inhaler for my congestion and breathing problems. He also prescribed naproxen for my knee and shoulder pain claiming that it was just inflammation. In addition, he wanted me to starting seeing a physical therapist.

I started getting care from Baker Chiropractic and Wellness

around the end of October or beginning of November. I didn't know much about chiropractic care before I started here and I was definitely skeptical. I had heard so many rumors that it was just a doctor cracking your back to get money and that it really didn't work. My mother didn't want me to be seen by a chiropractor. She wanted me to physical therapy at first.

Ever since I have been receiving chiropractic care, I feel a lot healthier in general. I am back to lifting and working out 100%. I even tell my friends and family members that chiropractic care is one of the best things for my health that I have invested into. I feel like I have more energy and that I'm in the best shape I have ever been in.

Without chiropractic care, I would probably be seeing a physical therapist and taking inflammation medication. I have nothing against physical therapy but physical therapy can only do so much in strengthening muscles around my joints. I would have continued to train as I do every day and that would have lead to me getting some type of surgery in the future.

I would and do recommend others with similar health problems to get checked out by Baker Chiropractic and Wellness. Like I said, I have never experienced care from anywhere like the care I receive here. They sat me down and opened my eyes by teaching me what was going on with my body and why I was having the pain.

The new patient orientation at Baker Chiropractic and Wellness is so eye opening and such a great learning experience. It has inspired me to become a chiropractor someday and help others avoid needless medications and surgery.

— **Terrence H.**

· · · · ·

61
Leg Pain

I have had extreme low back pain, hip pain and leg pain for well over ten years which greatly limited my normal, day-to-day activities.

In my search for help with my pain issues, I would have done just about anything to get relief!

My many visits to a local chiropractor and physicians proved futile. I endured various scans, tests and procedures only to realize that it was a complete waste of my time and effort. I was getting worse and could not even enjoy being a Dad to my son!

It was then that a co-worker told me about Dr. Patrick Baker at Baker Chiropractic and Wellness.

My first adjustment seemed to be somewhat painful but when I stood up, I quickly realized that my long term pain was GONE! I

By Dr. Paul Baker, Dr. Patrick Baker and Hundreds of Patients

was, and continue to be AMAZED at my ongoing progress!

No more pain when getting in and out of my vehicle. No more discomfort when sitting or driving for an extended period of time!

Now I can play with my son! My pain is gone! It really is!

Thank you Dr. Baker and staff!

You have all been God's hand extended to me!

— **Andrew S.**

• • • • •

I have been seeing Dr. Paul Baker and Dr. Garrett Knuckles for about six months now and I am very happy with the results.

For the past five years I have had extreme pain in my lower back, legs and abdomen areas. I had seen about ten doctors over that period of time in the pain management, orthopedic and other specialists trying to come up with a solution to my problem. This was a very depressing and painful path for myself as well as my family but I was finally brought to Baker Chiropractic and Wellness.

This is the first time I didn't hear surgery or medication was going to be needed. Dr. Paul and Dr. Garrett both spent time with me not just adjusting but talking to me about ways to improve my situation. For the first time I felt like someone took a real interest in my health and was trying to find a solution. I am not 100% yet but I am more than 50% better than I was six months ago.

The best part about my entire experience at Baker Chiropractic and Wellness is the actual staff. They are friendly, caring, and always courteous to my needs.

I will certainly recommend Baker Chiropractic and Wellness to my family and friends. Two thumbs up!

— Steve C.

• • • • •

There are a couple of things you should know about me before I give you my "testimony" about my experiences with Dr. Patrick Baker.

1. My grandmother nicknamed me "Bea" because I started walking at 8 months. I have never stopped....

2. I am a firm believer in the fact that if possible, our bodies will heal themselves without medicine to mask the pain or surgery to "fix" it, IF given the proper nutrition, exercise and rest.

Now to my story...

After a long and fun three-day weekend with my girlfriends, where I drove 11 hours in three days, wore a new pair of tennis shoes while walking endless hours to shop, and slept in a bed I was not used to, I woke up two days later with severe pain down my left leg and across my back.

Now, I am not talking "take a Tylenol and go to bed" kind of pain. I could not stand up straight, could not lay down in any comfortable position, could not walk more than 10 feet and when I moved, I literally cried out in agony. I had double knee replacements (both at the same time) six years ago and the pain from that did not match what I was experiencing.

After reading some on-line exercises and treatments and trying to "doctor" myself for a week, I called Dr. Baker, whom I had seen several years ago after an auto accident. I went in for a consultation and X-ray to see what could possibly be the problem. I could barely stand up long enough to get the X-rays taken.

Dr. Baker looked at the results and did some muscle stimulation therapy and ultrasound and then adjusted my back. I felt great! But it only lasted for about 15 minutes. By the time I walked to my car and pulled myself in the seat (my husband was driving me), the severe pain was back. I had made appointments to come back daily to see Dr. Baker. The pain was horrible and I couldn't sleep, stand, sit, lay or anything without discomfort—no, that is too mild—without excruciating pain! I cancelled Thanksgiving off at my house and had done NO Christmas shopping!

I went back to Dr. Baker day after day, six days a week. After the 2nd week of treatments, well-meaning friends and family members began to direct me to websites and forward me phone numbers of surgeons in the area. I continued to see Dr. Baker. By the middle of the third week, now the beginning of December, my pain level was at a 9 most of the time (down from what I considered to be an 11 on a scale of 1-10!) The pain in my left leg was so severe that I began to think I had bone cancer or a break in the femur of which I was unaware! I was in tears when I talked to Dr. Baker that day. He just told me to "hang in there; it will get better."

I did begin to feel a tiny, miniscule bit of relief after leaving his office. Generally for about 60-90 minutes my pain level would be bearable. I can't say I was without pain at all. My leg, even if not aching like a toothache, still hurt all the time. By week four, I could actually see some progress. I began to be able to work a bit, move around and get in and out of my car with relative ease. I continued to see Dr. Baker 4-6 times a week.

By the week before Christmas, now a full 6 weeks had passed, I could function with minimal pain until around 6 p.m. By that time I was in the chair the rest of the night. My husband took a photo of me sitting on a stool cooking dinner because I couldn't stand that long at the stove!

Little by little, the pain was gone from adjustment time till close to bed time—12-14 hours at a stretch. I had a trip coming in January to a sales conference and I was concerned about getting around at the airport and then walking around for three days at a conference. But my pain began to diminish rapidly by Christmas. I wasn't ready to dance a jig, but certainly a waltz!

Now I have been seeing Dr. Baker for nearly two months. The pain in my back and down my leg is nearly gone; the numbness in my left thigh is almost normal, but still tingles a bit. I can walk, stand, move and even go to the grocery store without worrying about "making it through." I am now down to twice a week and I will continue to see Dr. Baker, or one of his associates, weekly. I don't know for how long, maybe forever, I just know I NEVER want to be in that much pain again. I am leaving for my conference tomorrow!

I remember seeing the poster on the wall in his West Chester clinic of the progression of life, from baby to adult, then stooping, walking with a walker and in a wheel chair. I literally saw myself in that poster and know without his help, I would probably be on a surgeon's table by now. His Maximized Living is my next step and I know that with the proper nutrition, exercise and rest, my 62 year old body can once again "dance a jig!"

Thanks Dr. Patrick Baker, Dr. Brock Frear and the entire staff at Baker Chiropractic and Wellness. You are all amazing!

— **Patricia S.**

．　．　．　．　．

I have been experiencing back and leg pain for more than six years. The medical and related therapy had not been able to solve the problems. My specialized doctor was considering back surgery, which my brother had done and he highly recommend that this be my last resort.

My wife and I were consulting with my friend and former neighbor (Don) on a landscaping item and he noticed that I could not stand for any length of time.

He suggested I schedule an appointment with Dr. Baker and his staff. Since I had x-rays and MRI scans, Dr. Baker reviewed them and suggested the proper treatment. I started that same day. Dr. Baker and his staff have performed massages, electrical stimulation and chiropractic adjustments, which have solved many of my problems. I had one emergency problem, Dr. Baker and his staff handled it immediately without any advanced appointment.

If you have problems, please do not wait. Dr. Baker and his staff are very professional in their chiropractic healing. A very friendly and great environment!

— Joe

• • • • •

I fell and all my weight was put on my right leg. The pain was so bad that I could not stand on my right leg. I had an MRI, sonogram, x-rays and plenty of pain pills. They didn't help at all.

My friend told me about Dr. Baker and I started going to him. Now, I can walk up and down stairs and no more pain pills!

I'm planning on using my new tread mill and playing golf again. Thank you for making me feel good – without pain pills.

— J. Denny

• • • • •

62
Lymphadenopathy

My name is Debbie and chiropractic care was way outside of my comfort zone. I mean, who wants to have their bones snapped, cracked, and popped (LOL-sounds like cereal). Not me!

But I had pain radiating from my right shoulder to my thumb, which by the way, was numb all the time. This pain was constant while standing, sitting or lying down.

Sleep, forget it, not happening! Did I mention I'm right handed and watching an active 3 yr old, a guarantee for chaos. Chaos causes stress which aggravates the pain, so I was stuck in a viscous cycle.

My husband saw Baker Chiropractic and Wellness on TV, explaining how to help reduce pain. He asked me to go and see if I could at least get some relief for my pain. I knew he meant well, but I asked him why he didn't go get his shoulder fixed first. (Me – a guinea pig – yeah right !)

He felt I was in worse shape as I had already been to 2 orthopedic doctors, given medication (which did not help) and the next step was exploratory surgery. That surgery was not guaranteed to give me any pain relief and came with a strong possibility of causing more problems with scar tissue. So he had me call that day. I figured it would take a long time to get in, but NO, they were able to get me in right away, just wonderful, NOT.

He even drove me there, just to make sure I went. (He knows me too well!) Calming but uplifting music was heard upon entering Baker Chiropractic and Wellness and yes, I did check, no broken bodies, WhooHoo!

The only thing I saw was smiling personnel with caring attitudes being encouraging. On top of that, you guessed it, hugs. I'm the Grouch when I'm in pain, like, leave me alone, don't look at me, don't talk to me and definitely, don't touch me. But our meeting with Dr Patrick Baker was different than what I expected. He was only concerned about getting me comfortable right away. Afterwards, he explained how to possibly get me back to a full PAIN FREE life. He sold my husband but hey, it's my body that will be disjointed; I did say pain makes me a Grouch. I had to decide, Dr Patrick or Pain?

Pain will motivate you to step out of your comfort zone. So I finally gave in; besides, I don't think my husband would let me go home without getting help.

So from October 21,2014 until now, Baker Chiropractic and Wellness has reduced or eliminated my pain and numbness, all without medication or surgery!

My shoulder, arm and thumb are back to 90%. Compression on spine, relieved, who knew that stopped migraines. Ribs not right, relieved, restored flexibility helped me with my grandbaby, tying my shoes, brushing my hair, reaching overhead, lots of everyday basic movements.

Chiropractic Adjustments (new word for me) help without hurting and the results are a better life. Adjustments are needed to return your body to its rightful alignment. I have gone to Dr. Patrick Baker, Dr. Joe Fields and Dr. Kelly Duffner to be adjusted, all with good results. It is rare today to like all the doctors in one practice, so I feel blessed.

December 2014 saw my husband coming here for his frozen shoulder which was at 15% flexibility, but now is around 80%.

Soon after talking to Dr. Patrick about how our 3 yr old grandson's doctor and surgeon were leaving his walnut-size lymph nodes alone until he turned 5, our grandson started seeing Dr Kelly Duffner in early 2015. The lymph nodes are now pea size.

Gavin loves going so much that whenever we drive in that direction, he is ready to go. He doesn't understand waiting your turn, so when we arrive, he climbs up on the bed and lays down waiting for Dr. Kelly to FIX him. I tried to explain ADJUSTMENTS to him, but he told me, Dr. Kelly doesn't ADJUST clothes, he FIXES bones. He loves Dr. Kelly and the tickle hammer.

Recently, our skeptical daughter started coming due to numbness in her shoulder and neck pain. Let's just say, she never misses her regular visits to Baker Chiropractic and Wellness.

Family doctors are needful and do well, but for this family it will be after our Chiropractic Care. There are no worries as we know that we'll be directed to our family doctor when needed.

Thank you Baker Chiropractic and Wellness family, (Dr. Patrick, Dr. Joe, Dr. Kelly, Jackie, Danielle and John), for your great care now and for many years ahead.

— **Debbie B.**

— **Tom B.**

— **Gavin (Grandson)**

• • • • •

63
Lymph Nodes

My name is Debbie and chiropractic care was way outside of my comfort zone. I mean, who wants to have their bones snapped, cracked, and popped (LOL-sounds like cereal). Not me !

But I had pain radiating from my right shoulder to my thumb, which by the way, was numb all the time. This pain was constant while standing, sitting or lying down.

Sleep, forget it, not happening! Did I mention I'm right handed and watching an active 3 yr old, a guarantee for chaos. Chaos causes stress which aggravates the pain, so I was stuck in a viscous cycle.

My husband saw Baker Chiropractic and Wellness on TV, explaining how to help reduce pain. He asked me to go and see if I could at least get some relief for my pain. I knew he meant well, but I asked him why he didn't go get his shoulder fixed first. (Me – a guinea pig – yeah right !)

He felt I was in worse shape as I had already been to 2 orthopedic doctors, given medication (which did not help) and the next step was exploratory surgery. That surgery was not guaranteed to give me any pain relief and came with a strong possibility of causing more problems with scar tissue. So he had me call that day. I figured it would take a long time to get in, but NO, they were able to get me in right away, just wonderful, NOT.

He even drove me there, just to make sure I went. (He knows me too well!) Calming but uplifting music was heard upon entering Baker Chiropractic and Wellness and yes, I did check, no broken bodies, WhooHoo!

The only thing I saw was smiling personnel with caring attitudes being encouraging. On top of that, you guessed it, hugs. I'm the Grouch when I'm in pain, like, leave me alone, don't look at me, don't talk to me and definitely, don't touch me. But our meeting with Dr Patrick Baker was different than what I expected. He was only concerned about getting me comfortable right away. Afterwards, he explained how to possibly get me back to a full PAIN FREE life. He sold my husband but hey, it's my body that will be disjointed; I did say pain makes me a Grouch. I had to decide, Dr Patrick or Pain?

Pain will motivate you to step out of your comfort zone. So I finally gave in; besides, I don't think my husband would let me go home without getting help.

So from October 21,2014 until now, Baker Chiropractic and Wellness has reduced or eliminated my pain and numbness, all without medication or surgery!

My shoulder, arm and thumb are back to 90%. Compression on spine, relieved, who knew that stopped migraines. Ribs not right, relieved, restored flexibility helped me with my grandbaby, tying my shoes, brushing my hair, reaching overhead, lots of everyday basic movements.

Chiropractic Adjustments (new word for me) help without hurting and the results are a better life. Adjustments are needed to return your body to its rightful alignment. I have gone to Dr. Patrick Baker, Dr. Joe Fields and Dr. Kelly Duffner to be adjusted, all with good results. It is rare today to like all the doctors in one practice, so I feel blessed.

December 2014 saw my husband coming here for his frozen shoulder which was at 15% flexibility, but now is around 80%.

Soon after talking to Dr. Patrick about how our 3 yr old grandson's doctor and surgeon were leaving his walnut-size lymph nodes alone until he turned 5, our grandson started seeing Dr Kelly Duffner in early 2015. The lymph nodes are now pea size.

Gavin loves going so much that whenever we drive in that direction, he is ready to go. He doesn't understand waiting your turn, so when we arrive, he climbs up on the bed and lays down waiting for Dr. Kelly to FIX him. I tried to explain ADJUSTMENTS to him, but he told me, Dr. Kelly doesn't ADJUST clothes, he FIXES bones. He loves Dr. Kelly and the tickle hammer.

Recently, our skeptical daughter started coming due to numbness in her shoulder and neck pain. Let's just say, she never misses her regular visits to Baker Chiropractic and Wellness.

Family doctors are needful and do well, but for this family it will be after our Chiropractic Care. There are no worries as we know that we'll be directed to our family doctor when needed.

Thank you Baker Chiropractic and Wellness family, (Dr. Patrick, Dr. Joe, Dr. Kelly, Jackie, Danielle and John), for your great care now and for many years ahead.

— **Debbie B.**
— **Tom B.**
— **Gavin (Grandson)**

• • • • •

64
Medical Doctors
Who Are Patients

When I first came to Dr. Paul at Baker Chiropractic, I could hardly walk because my back was in spasm. My residents and medical students had to push me around the hospital in a wheelchair! Using a well-rounded treatment approach including an absolutely painless adjustment, I was 30 percent better in just one visit. By the end of the week, I was walking upright and pain free. All without the need for anti-inflammatory medications, muscle relaxants, or pain pills!

— B. Masterson, MD

· · · · ·

It is my belief that Chiropractic Medicine is one of the misunderstood, underappreciated, and perhaps, effective treatment modalities available. I attribute my being able to remain off the "disabled list" to Dr. Paul Baker's remarkable clinical skill and knowledge.

— M. Heintzelman, PH.D.

· · · · ·

Before seeing Dr. Baker I was having pain in my neck and lower back that was radiating into my legs. My activity level and quality of life was quite limited. Now I still feel some occasional discomfort but the pain has subsided and I am now mobile enough to coach my daughter's basketball team and go shopping with my wife. I also really enjoy the family atmosphere in the office. Everyone is so friendly and remembers your name. This helps makes the total experience so pleasant.

— Dr. S. Thomas

· · · · ·

Just like Drs. Paul and Patrick Baker, I knew at a very young age that I wanted to care for people. I became a medical doctor dedicated to helping people prevent health problems from developing in the first place. As an OB/GYN who has cared for hundreds of expectant mothers and delivered their babies, pregnant women as well as their newborn children can benefit greatly from chiropractic care in the prevention and treatment of many ailments, disorders and diseases. Removing subluxations through chiropractic care enables people of all ages to maximize their health.

— M. Pelletier, M.D., C.C.N., F.A.C.O.G.

LaValle Metabolic Institute

Director of Functional Medicine

65
Migraines

I went from being an insurance adjuster denying chiropractic claims to becoming an advocate for chiropractic care. My migraine headaches have finally been healed after 20 years!

I was asked to see Dr. Baker by Mrs. Renee Courtney (Pitts). I was experiencing severe migraines for the last I'll say 20 years. In 1997 they were the worse I had

ever had. I was on several medicines and decided to get off them cold turkey. Of course the doctor tells you not to do this. So please don't go cold turkey. I got very ill. But to this day I do not take all that medicine any longer. I do still experience the migraines.

In 2010, I was fainting while driving and they thought I was having seizures. So the Dr. had tests ran and put me on medication even though the tests would be negative. Then I would faint sitting at my desk and now they would send me to a heart specialist and they put me on medication as well, test still negative. Every time that I would faint I would be referred to some other doctor and they would put me on a prescription and the results were endless.

I was talking to Mrs. Courtney and she asked me if I would go to Dr. Baker with her just to see what he did. I was so skeptical because I used to process claims back in the day and chiropractors were not considered doctors of health. So I was denying claims left and right.

After being there Dr. Baker told me that he could help me. Well of course this sounded great. I was impressed with the wellness care and no medicine was involved. I went for the treatment plan and was amazed how much my spine was out of line.

I started to go and to my surprise I was able to see (I mean that the pain had me all fogged up). Everything looked clearer than I could imagine. The migraine was not as severe as before. And I was heading towards improvement.

Well then Dr. Baker went on vacation. The headache came right back. You see I was not getting the treatment while he was gone. Now I can say that the adjustments I am receiving is truly helping me. I look forward to getting the adjustments and feeling better.

I only talk about what I know and I know that the adjustments really work for me. I will tell every person I know that is having pain to at least think about what the medicine is doing to your body. If you can have an adjustment and not put a foreign object in your body than take the latter.

Now it has been over a year and I feel great the headaches only comes back if I am not receiving the proper adjustments to keep my body in line.

I look forwarding to see everyone in the office. It has been an amazing journey. I love going where I can talk about the Lord and seeing what God is doing in this practice. I have seen people literally get out of wheel chairs and return to walking. Look at God operating in Dr. Baker and his practice to do his work.

Everyone at Dr. Baker's office, I would like to thank you for being so kind and helping me see that there is a better way to healthy living.

A Special Thanks to Dr. Patrick Baker (keep doing God's work).

In Christ,
— **Catherine R.**

• • • • •

I came to Baker Chiropractic and Wellness for severe migraines but I also have IBS and a history with RSD.

I've suffered with migraines for 11 years. In the past 2 to 3 years they've been more severe and increasingly constant to the point that I can't remember what it's like to not have a headache and to feel fully present and focused.

I've taken innumerable medications from the time I was 12 years old. I went through every migraine medicine out there and have gone through the gamut again in the past two years. I take 75mg TOPOMAX® daily (a seizure medication), 40mg RELPAX® with the onset of a migraine and I get 40 BOTOX®

injections every three months. My body keeps getting used to the medicine and I hate the side effects, so it's not ideal. I resorted to leaving my job and resting to try and heal quicker.

I couldn't enjoy anything I wanted to do – walking my dog, hiking or riding bikes with my husband. I can't count the number of wedding receptions we've had to leave early because of my migraines.

I sought chiropractic care 2 years ago, but the chiropractor I went to did not do corrective care and his approach had no results. When I first came to Baker Chiropractic and Wellness in September, I was very skeptical until I learned about their corrective care approach.

Today, I have hope again! My migraines are still healing but for the first time I feel like I'm on a team with my doctor. Dr. Joe (Fields) doesn't write prescriptions and say, "Be patient". He invests in the whole health of his patients and takes their healing personally. I love having a home regimen to work on outside of my adjustments. It's so different than popping pills and hoping something works.

If it weren't for Baker Chiropractic and Wellness, I would be seeing more doctors, filling more prescriptions and losing hope that I could ever escape the migraines. I constantly worry about how all the medications I've taken in the past will impact me in the long run.

Every doctor I've been to before now is trying to fix us from the outside in, but Baker Chiropractic and Wellness is looking at the inside first – where the problem starts. They are not just any chiropractor. They really invest in you and your whole health.

I can't recommend them highly enough!

— Claire B

• • • • •

In my line of business, validation of results means everything before calling something a success. In the case of my treatment at Baker Chiropractic, I have made significant enough progress where I can declare success!

I have been affected by migraine type headaches and separately with lower back issues for over 10 years. I learned to "deal" with both but each had gotten progressively worse to the point that it was time to seek help in resolving the problem. The headaches have been my clear focus since I was getting them 3 or even 4 times a week and they could get to levels bad enough that I could not function well.

I used to think my headaches were sinus related since I used to feel pain and pressure in my ear and sinus cavities of my cheek and around the eyes. I used to take a LOT of pseudoephedrine and either ibuprofen or acetaminophen. My first visit with the Baker's demonstrated to me that the cause was a subluxation that caused my muscles to tighten through my shoulders and neck, further affecting the other nerves. My first adjustment and treatment with Dr. Paul provided near immediate relief and showed me the real cause of my pain. Since that first visit 1-1/2 years ago Dr. Pat has gotten me to the point where a headache is a rare event for me and we can now concentrate on completely eliminating them for this cause. The other issue of my lower back pain from old injuries has been getting better and as long as I don't do anything to re-injure it, I am expecting it too, to be eliminated.

I really like receiving treatment at the Baker's. The whole staff makes you feel like part of a family and not just a patient. The Baker program with Maximized Living treats the whole person and not just chiropractic treatment. It really helps a patient to understand everything that affects the health and wellness of our bodies. It doesn't matter who treats you at Baker Chiropractic. Even though Dr. Pat has provided treatment for me the most, I have also been treated by Drs. Paul, Kelly, Garrett and Joe and I have felt the same high quality of care from each. The healing effects from electrotherapy and deep tissue massages have been very instrumental with the chiropractic treatments to get me to a higher functioning condition where I am now.

I am very glad I made the decision to come to Baker's and I feel like I am well on my way to correcting past injuries and eliminating my chronic painful conditions.

— **Patrick D.**

· · · · ·

During my junior year of high school I began to experience chronic migraines. These migraines occurred several times a day and resulted in me missing over a month of school as well as losing 15 pounds. The migraines could be caused by almost anything, limiting my activities and ability to do anything I enjoyed.

After doing research trying to find a cure for these monstrous headaches I found they could be offset by chiropractic alignment and relieving the stress in the neck. I made an appointment at Dr. Baker's office immediately and have been seeing him several times a week ever since.

As a result of Dr. Baker my migraines were reduced to once a week, to once a month, and are now almost completely gone.

My life has since returned back to its normal state and has also improved. I am able to go to the gym 5-6 times a week and have much more energy. I've also gained back all the weight I had lost.

I've never had an experience like I have at Baker Chiropractic. When I walk in the door I am greeted one a first name basis, asked how I am doing and am seen extremely quickly.

I am beyond thankful for what Bakers Chiropractic has done for me.

Thanks Dr. Baker!

— **Amir K.**

• • • • •

When I first came to Baker Chiropractic I had been having migraines 2-3 times a week for a little over 3 years.

I would go to my family care physician and she would prescribe the newest medication for migraines. I got tired of taking medications and the side effects they were causing. I was tired all of the time and the migraines were not subsiding. It was either make a change or live a life full of medications and migraines.

I had a friend that swore by chiropractic medicine and said they might be able to help my migraines, so why not try it? I had essentially stopped living my life because I was always suffering. When I would get a migraine I would have to go to bed, nothing would help.

The first time to the office Dr. Baker told me after the adjustment to stop my medications and see how I did. I was slightly skeptical, but that weekend was migraine free. I was astounded at the results of the first adjustment and continued to come in weekly.

I feel so much better, I don't have the migraines anymore, and I got a new start at a life I'd been missing. I cannot thank Baker Chiropractic enough for helping me!

— **Kristine S.**

· · · · ·

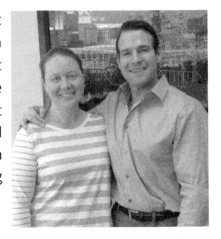

I decided to give chiropractic care a try in August of 2012. When I initially made the appointment to see Dr. Patrick Baker at the Fairfield Clinic, I had no idea that I would still be going a year and a half later or that it would turn out to be such a life-changing decision.

I originally made the appointment because I was having severe neck pain. I could not tilt my head from side to side and I would wake up from sleeping with constant headaches. After the spinal exam and X-ray results were in, I found out that I was suffering from a condition called Forward Head Posture. I have also suffered with migraines since I was thirteen, and Dr. Baker assured me that the chiropractic adjustments would help with those as well. I decided to proceed with Dr. Baker's treatment plan, and it was one of the best choices I have ever made.

After the first couple weeks of adjustments, I noticed a dramatic decrease in the level of neck pain I was experiencing. The constant headaches began to subside, and within a month, I was virtually pain free. And that was just the beginning. I also noticed that I was sleeping better and had more energy. And after just a couple months of care, the migraines became less frequent. I went from having migraines three to four times a month to just three to four times a year in the time I've been a patient.

I wish I would have known years ago how much chiropractic care could help with the migraines alone. I would have started going sooner. And I urge anyone reading this that does get migraines to give it a shot. It will really improve your quality of life, much more so than those triptans we all get when we tell our docs that we get migraines. As if the migraine itself isn't bad enough, we're prescribed pills that only work some of the time and leave us in a sleepy haze for three days afterwards. No thanks. I'll take a massage and an adjustment instead. At least then I know I'm treating the problem and not the symptom – as evidenced by the fact that I no longer get the migraines with any real frequency. And when I do get them, they are much less severe. I no longer take triptans to treat them. Or any prescription medicine, for that matter. Since I had been feeling so much better, I asked Dr. Baker to help me with stepping down off the antidepressant I had been prescribed three years ago because I had no lingering symptoms of depression and I felt like the meds were keeping me in a constant fog. He referred me to Dr. Theodore Cole at the Cole Center for Healing, and with their help, I was able to successfully step down of the medicine two months ago without any side effects. Except a little weight loss.

Which brings me to the bonus: since attending the Baker Chiropractic Total Food Makeover seminar in February of 2013 and slowly implementing the nutrition and fitness guidelines that were provided, I have lost 40 pounds. And I'm still losing!

That's what I have enjoyed so much about this whole experience. It has been nothing but positive, and the doctors and staff are truly invested in helping you achieve your health goals. They take the time to educate you and provide you with the tools that you need to succeed. I am grateful to all of them for their help and support. I don't even want to think about what my quality of life would be like right now had I not decided to seek chiropractic care. So if you're thinking about giving it a try, just go for it. It will be one of the best decisions you ever make.

— **Amanda G.**

· · · · ·

My teenage son awoke one morning with blurred vision and sensitivity to light. I attributed it to lack of sleep or too much "screen time", and insisted that he go to school. I also knew that we had a scheduled visit with an ophthalmologist in a few days. It had been nearly two years since his eyes had been checked and he was overdue for new lenses.

Not long after arriving at school, he reported to the nurse with a debilitating headache. I brought him home where he spent the rest of the day on the living room sofa in the dark. I took him to the pediatrician that evening. The pediatrician looked into his eyes with a scope and had him read an eye chart. We were sent directly to the emergency room of a Children's Hospital. After four hours and a phone call to a neurologist, the staff pediatrician looked into my son's eyes with a scope and had him read an eye chart. The consensus was that he had a migraine headache.

We pretty much suspected that, but I was concerned about the sudden onset of blurred vision, as it might indicate something was immediately going wrong in his brain, like a concussion, aneurysm tumor ... parents think like that, right?

We were relieved to finally be dismissed from the ER, with orders for my son to take a pain reliever and get a good night's sleep. If the headaches persisted, we should consult a neurologist who could prescribe a drug for migraine headaches.

331

The next morning, my son awoke with blurred vision, extreme sensitivity to light, and pain in the back of his head. The next day was another day on the sofa, taking pain relievers and no school.

Day three went pretty much the same way, except we made a visit to our chiropractor, Dr. Paul Baker. Dr. Paul told us that his C2 vertebrae was subluxated. After one adjustment, the relief was immediate. After two chiropractic treatments, neck traction with a Dakota cushion at home, good nutrition, sleep and back to drinking the recommended daily amount of water, my son's migraine headaches have not returned.

We continue our regular visits to Dr. Paul. He and the staff treat us like family. The care is genuine and the results are real. My son has new glasses, too. He likes to research topics on the internet. He learned that approximately 20% of teenagers are affected by migraine headaches. Drugs prescribed for migraines can have serious effects on the liver and heart. The ocular nerve that affects vision is located by the C2 vertebrae.

Poor posture from staring at a computer screen for long periods can cause subluxations in your spine. We are so grateful to have Dr. Baker straighten things out for us.

Drug free, real cures. That's what Baker Family Chiropractic is all about.

— **Kimberly F and son Jerry**

• • • • •

When I was seventeen years old I fractured my neck and two bones in my back. I was very lucky that I wasn't hurt worse than I was. I went through six months of being in a neck cast, 8 hours of surgery, and then six additional months of physical therapy. Pain was a daily issue for me. My muscles were so tight that I would constantly have migraines. I couldn't focus. There would be days that I would just shut the whole world out, and go to a dark quiet place just to find some sort of relief, but still there was none.

One day, my Mom told me to go to Dr. Baker since he has helped everyone in my family. I thought ok, I'll give it a try. Why not? That was the best decision I could have ever made. Within one week I could tell a difference. Within a month I was headache free.

Something that I never thought would happen. I could actually enjoy life again. I can't even put a price on that. Words cannot describe how grateful I am to Dr. Baker and his staff. They gave me my life back.

— **Brittany B.**

• • • • •

I began care at Baker Chiropractic and Wellness in early 2014 due to chronic headaches, migraines, and back pain. I had been plagued by headaches from the time I was a small child and chronic back pain for nearly a decade.

The migraines began roughly two years before I began my chiropractic care here. I was having between two and three migraines a week. As a mother of four children at that time, it certainly made daily life challenging. Exercise, diet and over-the-counter medications brought little relief and nothing lasting.

Shortly after receiving care at Baker Chiropractic and Wellness, I began to notice improvement. The chronic back pain had greatly diminished and within three months of starting my care, the headaches had ceased, except for the occasional stress or dehydration headache. The migraines also completely stopped with the exception of a monthly hormonal headache. Not only did I physically feel better, I felt better mentally and there was a noticeable energy increase.

I also received chiropractic care during my fifth pregnancy. Dr. Joe Fields helped my, at one point breach and at another point posterior, baby get into the right position. He also helped bring comfort to the normal pregnancy aches and is continuing to help now, six weeks postpartum, with my recovery.

I am extremely grateful for Dr. Joe and Baker Chiropractic and Wellness for their wonderful care and the gift of a healthy and more active life.

By Dr. Paul Baker, Dr. Patrick Baker and Hundreds of Patients

My daughter Anna also began her chiropractic care with Baker Chiropractic and Wellness in early 2014 due to headaches and cyclic vomiting syndrome.

She has dealt with headaches and cyclic vomiting from the time she was roughly two years of age. Hydration, diet modification, herbal supplementation, extra rest and over-the-counter medication offered no lasting relief. Traditional medicine can do little for cyclic vomiting, aside from treating the symptoms.

These issues greatly hindered Anna's ability to truly partake in activities that a young girl greatly enjoys. Activities such as sleepovers, camps and anything prohibiting a nap were very difficult and rare because overexertion and excitement could trigger an episode.

Once Anna began chiropractic care she experienced immediate relief from the plaguing headaches and a substantial decrease in the duration of an episode.

Now roughly a year later, Anna is almost completely free from the cyclic vomiting. Chiropractic care has greatly improved Anna's life and health, and we are forever grateful for Baker Chiropractic and Wellness and Dr. Joe Fields for their kind and tender care towards our sweet daughter.

I cannot recommend them enough, especially for the treatment of cyclic vomiting syndrome.

— Amberly W.

• • • • •

66
Multiple Sclerosis (MS)

Dear Dr. Baker and Staff - We have been regular patients at your Fairfield office for over ten years now and are very happy with our experiences there. You and your staff are always friendly and helpful in addition to efficient in administering effective treatments.

Cindy's experiences:

I was diagnosed with multiple sclerosis (MS) in the early 1990s and my mobility gradually decreased for several years. Physical therapy routines and medications helped to suspend my physical decline at a point where I have limited mobility (use wheelchair, walker, hand-holds, etc.). After finding physical therapy alone was not enough to maintain my mobility, I decided to try chiropractic therapy.

My neurologist is supportive of chiropractic treatment to manage the effects of MS, and I believe regular chiropractic treatments are allowing me to maintain my limited mobility by keeping the parts of my body I over-use or under-use in a flexible state rather than allowing them to atrophy.

I have been treated regularly by Dr. Baker for about 15 years now, and this has helped me maintain my mobility at a stable level. These regular treatments also help to avoid and provide relief from occasional bouts of sciatic nerve pain (probably indirectly associated with the MS). I believe it likely I would be confined to a wheelchair without these regular chiropractic treatments.

I have also observed a decrease in mobility with time when I am unable to receive my regular chiropractic treatments. I believe chiropractic treatments are making a significant difference in my quality of life with MS.

Tony's experiences:

I have always been fairly active. I used to play softball regularly, I bowl regularly, I coached outdoor sports for my sons, I golf occasionally and go on occasional fishing marathons, in addition to the normal yard work etc. associated with maintaining a home.

Previous to regular chiropractic treatment, I would periodically (1-2 times/year) experience painful and debilitating pinched nerve problems in my upper back/shoulder area. These were treated with muscle relaxing drugs before I began visiting Dr. Baker.

I have not experienced a single pinched nerve incident during the approximately 15 years I have been treated by Dr. Baker. This is amazing to me, and I am definitely happy with these results!

Thanks – and keep up the good work!

— Tony and Cindy D.

67
Neck Fusion

My name is Mary Ann and I am a patient of Dr. Patrick Baker. I have been with Dr. Patrick since August of 2014.

I first came to Baker Chiropractic and Wellness to seek relief from chronic pain in the lower back and lower extremities. I had been

experiencing pain, tingling, and numbness for several years and finally I decided it was time to seek help.

From the very first phone call to his office, up until today, I have been treated as if I were their only patient. Dr. Patrick and his capable staff are consummate professionals and have been such help to me. My initial consultation revealed that I had a pinched nerves and subluxations in the lower lumbar spine. A treatment plan was developed based on my x-rays.

I must admit, I never really knew anything about chiropractic care and was somewhat skeptical. Boy was I wrong! I feel so much better in all areas of my body. What I learned was that not only could Dr. Patrick help my low back pain, but he could also help me with my neck pain despite the fact that I had a neck fusion surgery ten years ago.

I was always under the misunderstanding that since my neck was fused, I could never be treated by a chiropractor. Lo and behold, I can and my neck hasn't felt this great in years! I owe it to Dr. Baker and his team of knowledgeable professionals.

Dr. Patrick also treats my hands for carpel tunnel and my toes for hammertoe problems. Who knew?!? Fingers and toes as well.

The best part of it all is that Dr. Patrick, all of the other doctors, and the whole healing team really cares about you and your recover. They teach you complete wellness and encourage healthy lifestyles. The entire atmosphere during your visit is very positive and rewarding!

— Mary Y.

· · · · ·

68
Neck and
Shoulder Pain

In the spring of 2017, I started a project in my backyard. While working on that project I injured my right shoulder.

At first I didn't think much of it, although I couldn't raise my arm above my shoulder. I thought it was just soreness and getting older catching up to me.

The problem persisted for a few more weeks and became very painful if I moved my shoulder in almost any direction. It was getting worse rather than getting better and I was also having trouble sleeping with this condition. I was stubborn and let it go for a few months, just dealing with the pain. I finally couldn't take it any longer.

By Dr. Paul Baker, Dr. Patrick Baker and Hundreds of Patients

After experiencing going through hernia surgery the year before and dealing with my insurance and a high deductible, I decided to try chiropractor care instead of going to see my regular doctor and an orthopedic doctor.

At first I was a little skeptical. After my first couple visits and my examination/evaluation by Dr. Garrett Knuckles, I was still a little skeptical but thought it best to give it a try. Man was I glad I did.

I was given a plan to have 3 adjustments per week for 3 months. After the first couple weeks I made some decent progress and was very happy with how things were going. Dr. Knuckles had told me that shoulders were tricky at the beginning and that it will take a while to see some good progress.

The next couple weeks, honestly and frankly, were not so good. I didn't think I was making any more progress, and at times thought I was going backwards. The range of motion was staying the same and the pain had actually increased a little. Dr. Knuckles could tell I was getting a little irritated and depressed. He reminded me again this is part of the process, it will get better. Well he was right.

The last 3 or 4 weeks of my treatments I have seen steady improvement in range of movement and very little pain. I almost feel back to normal now at the end of my treatments, having almost full range of motion and no pain.

Dr. Garrett Knuckles and the entire staff at Baker Chiropractic and Wellness were very professional and kind, always making every visit a positive experience. I will recommend them to all my friends and family and will definitely be back for regular treatments.

— **Tim V.**

• • • • •

"Before going to seek treatment from Dr. Garrett Knuckles at Baker Chiropractic and Wellness, I was experiencing neck pain, lower back pain, sharp pain in my left arm and I was walking with a limp. I was also experiencing numbness in my hips which was keeping me up at night.

Dr. Garrett started me on a regiment of adjustments and in as little as four months I am now able to sleep through the night, I am practically pain free, and my limp no longer exists!

My life is so much better now thanks to Dr. Garrett and his staff!"

— **Norma S.**

• • • • •

Dear Dr. Patrick ,

I just want to give you a great big Hallelujah shout out for your expertise. Baker Chiropractic and Wellness Center has truly been a Godsend. I originally visited your Fairfield office due to a car accident in March 2013. I was in excruciating pain and I was provided immediate relief through your specialized chiropractic care for my back, neck, and shoulder pain.

I gained such relief & energy that I was able to return to enjoying quality of life again after just a few weeks of treatment. I felt so alive after completing your recommended treatment plan in June

2013, that I decided to not return for maintenance care as you had so sincerely suggested.

Well, while on vacation In July 2016, I woke up in excruciating pain to the point that I literally could not walk or bare any weight on my lower back to left buttock and leg. The pain was radiating through my left leg to foot and I was not able to walk without assistance of someone.

As recommended by my primary physician, I was taking steroid pain medicine around the clock every 4-6 hours only to get little if any relief. Upon my return home the pain had magnified to an off the chart level. Our family physician ordered an MRI which disclosed that I had two (2) pinched nerves pressing against a bulging herniated disc. I was referred to a neurosurgeon for further evaluation regarding the results of the MRI. After a consultation meeting with a surgeon, I was advised that an epidural injection should relieve the excruciating pain; after which I would be reevaluated for possible back surgery. I had the injection on August 5, 2016, which relieved the excruciating pain but the pain returned after a few days. I still was not able to sit, stand, or walk without the assistance of someone. I was basically restricted to mostly lying down while taking pain medicine.

At the persistence of my husband, I called Baker Chiropractic and Wellness on August 9th and was advised to come into the office the next day. I entered the office with tears from the severity of the pain I was still experiencing. Dr Patrick immediately performed spine adjustments and manipulations of which I felt immediate relief. I continued to see Dr. Patrick three (3) times a week and each day I became stronger with less pain. I was sitting, standing, and walking again on my own and enjoying my quality of life again! However, I was not able to continue recommended maintenance visits due to insurance policy demanding that I seek physical therapy instead of chiropractic care.

Thus, I was forced to go through physical therapy from September through December 2016. The therapy however was not as effective as the healing adjustments/spinal manipulative therapy that I received by Dr. Patrick and his team. But as fate would have it; while sitting at a red traffic light On April 21, 2017, I was abruptly rear-ended by an oncoming car. So once again, I returned to receive care from Dr. Patrick and Baker Chiropractic and Wellness Center.

I am writing this testimony in June 2017, with such appreciation for the special care and attention I have received from Dr. Patrick and his staff. I am an advocate believer of holistic healing and can say that I received such healing by following through with the recommended spine adjustments and manipulations along with other therapeutic treatments for pain management as performed and/or suggested you.

So again, a great BIG Hallelujah shout out to you Dr. Patrick and your love for people and your expertise in chiropractic healing through appropriately applied spinal and other body adjustments, manipulations, etc as deem necessary for a complete outcome of Wellness.

Thank you so much!!!

— Narkittia D.

· · · · ·

I first visited Baker Chiropractic and Wellness about 7 months ago. I suffered with chronic vertigo and neck problems for over a year.

My ENT physician sent me for extensive medical testing. From his recommendation, I attended vestibular therapy at the hospital and began taking medications. These treatments helped very little.

I did some research and decided to try chiropractic care. I was a bit skeptical.

I met Dr. Kelly (Duffner) on my first visit to Baker Chiropractic and Wellness. He took x-rays and explained the problems with my neck and spine. He was very confident that chiropractic treatment would help me.

After two weeks of treatment, I knew my symptoms were diminishing. I first noticed that my neck no longer hurt. Also, my vertigo symptoms were less intense.

My treatment continued, and after a couple of months, I felt quite a bit better. Treatment at Baker Chiropractic and Wellness has allowed me to return to work and I continue to make progress.

Chiropractic care is the only thing that has helped relieve my symptoms. I no longer need medications.

Dr. Kelly Duffner and Dr. Patrick Baker have been great throughout my treatment and I am grateful for their help.

— Jason H.

. . . . .

I started care here at Baker Chiropractic and Wellness less than three months ago.

I was living with low back pain for five years and severe neck pain from a car accident.

It was painful to ride my horse and pick-up my grandchildren.

To deal with the pain, I used Motrin and anti-inflammatory medications.

I was skeptical about chiropractic care at first. I didn't really believe in it. I thought it was just popping and moving bones.

After the care I have received at Baker Chiropractic and Wellness, I was able to take a 4-hour flight with absolutely no pain. I can also now ride my horse again for hours with no problem.

If I would not have come here, I would still be in pain.

I recommend that anyone who has back pain or neck pain like I did to come here and get evaluated.

— Colleen A.

. . . . .

I came to Baker Chiropractic and Wellness in August with pinched nerves, low back pain, sciatica, neck pain, and fibromyalgia. These problems had been going on for 4 to 5 months and prevented me from doing yoga, exercising and living my everyday life.

Prior to coming here, I had been taking over-the-counter medications to treat my symptoms but found no relief.

The chiropractic care I receive at Baker Chiropractic and Wellness is essential for me. It has relieved my pain and increased my mobility, all without having to use over-the-counter or prescription medications.

If not for Baker Chiropractic and Wellness, I would be in a lot of pain today. I definitely recommend this to anyone. The results I have seen are very promising!

— **Nita P.**

• • • • •

I had neck and lower back pain and have not experienced any symptoms since. It was a great experience. I'll look for referrals for you. Hope to see you soon. We're trying to have another baby, so when I get pregnant, I'll call you for adjustments (treatments). Thanks!

— **Melissa C.**

• • • • •

I was having neck and shoulder pain that was chronic. I already knew Dr. Worthington from his high school years. He seems very knowledgeable and from past experience I knew chiropractic would help. Now the pain is less severe. I would recommend anyone I find with similar symptoms because it seems to be helping me.

— **Brenda S.**

• • • • •

My name is Marlene and I was at the point of thinking "If this is what growing old is like, it's no fun!"

I had neck pain and back problems for 20+ years. I always felt sick and was unable to look up or turn my head.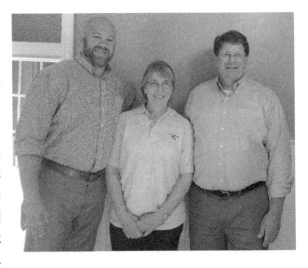
I couldn't do things I enjoy like gardening or slow dancing. I couldn't hug anyone or turn my head to chat with someone.

I started chiropractic care as a last chance before having to undergo neck surgery. When I started to see signs of recovery with chiropractic care, I knew this was the answer and I wanted total and complete recovery.

Not only did I get mobility back with my neck and back but I found I could now lay on my right side without immediate dizziness.

Recently, my family doctor said I had arthritis in my wrists. Oh my aching hands. Dr. Joe Fields took a look and fixed them with just one adjustment. He takes care of my wrists every week now. No more aching!

After chiropractic care at Baker Chiropractic and Wellness, I can now:

- Look up
- Hug people
- Lay down however I want without dizziness
- Turn my head from side-to-side
- Hold my head up

I also had no idea chiropractic care could fix my aching hands and in the last two weeks, I can breath with my mouth closed. No more snoring!

I got my life back. I can live because I can move!

My name is Tim and I had been struggling with headaches, lower back pain and hip problems for a few years. I was diagnosed with osteoarthritis and given pain killers for the hip pain. I eventually had both hips replaced and I couldn't do much of anything.

The chiropractic care I have received at Baker Chiropractic and Wellness gives me energy, mobility and just makes me feel better overall. I would not be able to work 12+ hour days without chiropractic care. I am also sick far less and haven't had a case of the flu since coming here.

— Marlene and Tim M.

• • • • •

I was bothered by stiff necks and having a lot of trouble with neck pain and headaches. To treat my pain and discomfort I was using ice packs and taking a lot of Advil.

The stiffness and pain made it difficult to do everyday activities. I couldn't even clean my house without having to stop and lay down for awhile. I also like to golf but every time I would go golfing, I would have neck stiffness afterwards.

I put up with the pain and stiffness for over three years. I just dealt with it but I knew something needed to change. I couldn't keep living my life this way.

Prior to coming to Baker Chiropractic and Wellness, I didn't know anything about chiropractic care and how or why it works. In fact, I was very skeptical. However, after years of neck stiffness and pain, it was finally time to do something about it.

Today, I have no more neck stiffness, no more neck pain

and no more headaches because of the chiropractic care I have received here. I can even go golfing now without having to deal with stiffness and discomfort.

If I would have not come to Baker Chiropractic and Wellness, I am sure I would still be dealing with the pain and not living the life I wanted to live.

Would I recommend Baker Chiropractic and Wellness to someone who is dealing with stiff necks, neck pain and headaches? Absolutely! In fact, I tell everyone about this place, how they need to learn about chiropractic care and why it can help them get out of pain.

Thank you!

— Priscilla R.

• • • • •

I first stepped foot into Baker Chiropractic because of severe pain radiating in my neck.

I have suffered from recurring whiplash caused from bus accidents as a child that would flare up three to four times a year. I was used to experiencing the pain. But this last flare up wouldn't go away and practically debilitated me.

Three weeks later, the stabbing and throbbing pains made it

difficult to work, stand, sit, and impossible to drive or sleep. Then I met the great people at Baker Chiropractic and Wellness.

Dr. Brock (Frear) took me under his wing and I saw results within a few visits. He took the time to explain his evaluation of my x rays and to show me the subluxations in my spine that were the source of my pain.

In addition to the neck misalignment, Dr. Brock showed me how my hips were also out of alignment. I told him it was probably because I was babying a hurt knee. He replied that my knee was hurting because my hips were offset. He also commented on the fact that he would have thought I had issues with sciatica. My mouth dropped open as I admitted I did have on again/off again sciatic pain.

One adjustment later and I could definitely see a marked difference, not only in my neck but also in my knee. I had more range of motion in my neck, a decrease in pain, I could finally sleep at night, not to mention that I could climb stairs like a normal person again. (side note: I was not at the time suffering from sciatica so I don't know if that was solved or not – but with everything else that improved, I have no doubt that it has as well). After a couple of weeks, I felt like the old me... but better.

It's a joy to go to Baker Chiropractic and Wellness. Not only do I know that I'm correcting my health issues but also the warm and friendly atmosphere is welcoming and makes it a joy to be there. I love the holistic approach and the positivity that radiates the entire practice.

The addition of the massage therapy has helped heal the aches and pains and further preps my muscles and joints to accept the adjustments. And the home therapy gives me the tools to aid me to keep my back healthy.

Dr. Brock and all his staff have a passion for the work they are doing. They each have their own personal story to tell on how chiropractic care, specifically from Baker Chiropractic and Wellness, has enriched their lives and made their health better. It's refreshing to see people love the work they are doing....to the point where Dr. Brock says this isn't work for him and that he sees it as his joy/mission to help all of us live a happier, healthier life.

I, for one, am greatly appreciative.

I'm a true believer in Chiropractic Care from Baker Chiropractic and Wellness. I came to Baker Chiropractic to alleviate my neck pain but also found the cure for my knee and sciatic pain as well, not to mention making my other internal organs healthier. Life can't get better than that!

— **Patricia B.**

• • • • •

Thank God for my son DeJuan for referring me to Dr. Paul Baker. Having more than 30 years of internalizing stress in a negative way, I've had constant pain in my neck, shoulders, left arm and low back.

Within 60 days of seeing Dr. Paul, my pain has decreased and my posture has improved tremendously.

I am also stronger mentally, spiritually and physically. I can even breathe better.

God's grace has given me the Power to take charge and control of my life. I have a better understanding and perspective of the benefits of the chiropractic profession. It has enabled me to heal emotionally and exercise better stress management.

I am feeling empowered and I am better – that's what's important.

Love You, God Bless You and glad we are Family.

— Berdina D.

• • • • •

My name is Mary Ann and I am a patient of Dr. Patrick Baker. I have been with Dr. Patrick since August of 2014.

I first came to Baker Chiropractic and Wellness to seek relief from chronic pain in the lower back and lower extremities. I had been experiencing pain, tingling, and numbness for several years and finally I decided it was time to seek help.

From the very first phone call to his office, up until today, I have been treated as if I were their only patient. Dr. Patrick and his capable staff are consummate professionals and have been such help to me. My initial consultation revealed that I had a pinched nerves and subluxations in the lower lumbar spine. A treatment plan was developed based on my x-rays.

I must admit, I never really knew anything about chiropractic care and was somewhat skeptical. Boy was I wrong! I feel so much better in all areas of my body. What I learned was that not only could Dr. Patrick help my low back pain, but he could also help me with my neck pain, despite the fact that I had a neck fusion surgery ten years ago.

I was always under the misunderstanding that since my neck was fused, I could never be treated by a chiropractor. Lo and behold, I can and my neck hasn't felt this great in years! I owe it to Dr. Baker and his team of knowledgeable professionals.

Dr. Patrick also treats my hands for carpel tunnel and my toes for hammertoe problems. Who knew?!? Fingers and toes as well.

The best part of it all is that Dr. Patrick, all of the other doctors, and the whole healing team really cares about you and your recover. They teach you complete wellness and encourage healthy lifestyles. The entire atmosphere during your visit is very positive and rewarding!

— Mary Y.

· · · · ·

I would like to start off by saying it is a blessing to have Dr. Brock Frear in my life.

The injuries to my body probably started back in high school when I had a blow to the head from a sign falling from the ceiling in a grocery store where I was working. I was checked out by the doctor and they told me that I had minor injuries, but I had to file for worker's compensation. I couldn't turn my head to the left from this injury, but by being a teenager, you just go with the flow until the pain goes away.

As I got older and into my mid-30's I noticed that I was having slight pain throughout my shoulders, but everyone told me that it was stress from everyday life challenges. Things seemed to get worse as years went on. I would try every over-the-counter medicine for pain and it would help for a minute and then the pain would start back up. I tried ice packs and warm compress, but nothing seemed to take the pain away.

Last summer, I had an incident where I fell out of the tub on my left side and hit hard. I was so lucky that I didn't break anything. Then, August of the same year, I was in a car accident, and the driver hit me on the left side of my car so that just added fuel to the fire.

The pain was getting so bad that I had no energy to do anything. My body always felt like I had a thousand tons of bricks on my shoulders. I would put a smile on my face at work just to make it through the day, but when I got home, the only thing I wanted to do was lay down. It was to the point where my daughter would want me to take her shopping and I didn't have the energy to even do that.

One day I was at work and my co-worker told me about Baker Chiropractic and Wellness. I said I didn't want to go because I've only heard bad things about chiropractors and I don't want to be worse than I am now. She said just go talk with them and see what they say.

So I made an appointment and went through all the procedures and was in shock of the damage on my neck, spine and hips. I started to cry and Dr. Brock told me that he would get me back to normal.

So, I started my routine and still wasn't a believer in this chiropractic stuff, but as weeks went on, I could feel my body starting to change. Then after a few months, I could feel the energy coming back, and I could start to do more things with my daughter. Now, I feel myself walking taller and everything is going back in alignment like it's supposed to be.

After 36 visits, I saw my x-rays and was amazed at the outcome. I was so happy I had to hug Dr. Brock twice and told him thank you so much for getting me back in the groove of things to where I could function. Again, I'm so happy to have him in my life!"

— **Tammy B.**

· · · · ·

I couldn't move my neck and was overweight by more than 30 pounds. I didn't feel very good about myself as a person.

Now, I feel 100% better. I also believe chiropractic care is so much better than traditional medicine. If doctors in traditional medical practices approached their careers, their practices and most importantly their patients with the same attitude and work ethic as Dr. Baker, my attitude might be different.

Thank you Dr. Baker for being there for me and providing a much needed change in my life.

— **D. Krause**

· · · · ·

I came to see Dr. Baker because I was having trouble with my neck. I sit all day at a computer and my fingers in my right hand were going numb. I knew from past chiropractic care from another doctor the problem I was experiencing was from my neck. After several adjustments I was feeling so much better. While talking to Dr. Baker he told me that he could help me with my headaches and shoulder pain. This was something I thought I would have to live with the rest of my life.

My headaches were so frequent my primary care Doctor was having me log them so we could try to figure out what was triggering them. After several adjustments I am happy to say I am not suffering from them anymore.

My shoulders were so rounded forward I did not realize how bad they were. Now with Dr. Bakers help they are almost back to normal and my posture is so much better.

I like the way Dr. Baker takes into account the whole body. I came in for one problem and he has helped me so much more. I can't thank Dr. Baker and his staff enough for helping me feel better and have a better quality of life.

— J. Johnson

• • • • •

Ever since I started being a patient of Dr. Baker, he has helped me out so much. I have been a patient for about three months now and ever since I have felt great. I first came in with neck and lower back pains but as each week goes on, I feel better and better.

Dr. Baker and his team always welcome me no matter what, which also adds on the making me feel so much better.

I always tell people with pain to "Go see Dr. Baker and experience the benefits Baker Chiropractic gives all of their patients!"

— **Ratri R.**

• • • • •

I wanted to take a moment to chronicle my story of healing and ongoing restoration.

A year ago, February 2014, I called Dr. Baker's office out of desperation. I was in incredible neck pain and had already been to my primary care doctor who referred me to a neck and back specialist with the idea I would be heading for surgery.

So, with little hope... but lots of pain, I figured I'd try anything to ease my pain. My thought at the time was even if it would be temporary; I would see a chiropractor just until I could schedule a consultation and surgery (there was at least a month wait for an appointment).

I was definitely a skeptic... in fact, my normal reaction to chiropractor care would be mockery! Doc Baker said, "skeptics make the best patients". I didn't know at that point how true that statement would be!

After a few visits to Doctor Baker, I was feeling remarkably better. After a few weeks I canceled my appointments with the surgeon and in a few more weeks felt almost as good as new.

Today I go back a few times a month for maintenance adjustments and believe a healthy spine leads to a healthy life. I couldn't really believe how quickly I had felt better and despite by skepticism, how much I now believed in this practice.

I am often amazed at how much better I feel from something I was once so skeptical about. I'm glad I wasn't too stubborn to make that phone call and have an open mind because it is one of the best decisions I've ever made.

And, finally, anyone who has ever visited would be able to tell you: The positive energy and hope exuded by every employee and most patients is contagious and uplifting. They are definitely, "Healing Spines, One Day at a Time" but they are also doing so with an eternal purpose and uplifting people's lives in general when they do it.

— **Glen G.**

· · · · ·

My name is Debbie and chiropractic care was way outside of my comfort zone. I mean, who wants to have their bones snapped, cracked, and popped (LOL-sounds like cereal). Not me!

But I had pain radiating from my right shoulder to my thumb, which by the way, was numb all the time. This pain was constant while standing, sitting or lying down.

Sleep, forget it, not happening! Did I mention I'm right handed and watching an active 3 yr old, a guarantee for chaos. Chaos causes stress which aggravates the pain, so I was stuck in a viscous cycle.

My husband saw Baker Chiropractic and Wellness on TV, explaining how to help reduce pain. He asked me to go and see if I could at least get some relief for my pain. I knew he meant well, but I asked him why he didn't go get his shoulder fixed first. (Me – a guinea pig – yeah right !)

He felt I was in worse shape as I had already been to 2 orthopedic doctors, given medication (which did not help) and the next step was exploratory surgery. That surgery was not guaranteed to give me any pain relief and came with a strong possibility of causing more problems with scar tissue. So he had me call that day. I figured it would take a long time to get in, but NO, they were able to get me in right away, just wonderful, NOT.

He even drove me there, just to make sure I went. (He knows me too well!) Calming but uplifting music was heard upon entering Baker Chiropractic and Wellness and yes, I did check, no broken bodies, WhooHoo!

The only thing I saw was smiling personnel with caring attitudes being encouraging. On top of that, you guessed it, hugs. I'm the Grouch when I'm in pain, like, leave me alone, don't look at me, don't talk to me and definitely, don't touch me. But our meeting with Dr Patrick Baker was different than what I expected. He was only concerned about getting me comfortable right away. Afterwards, he explained how to possibly get me back to a full PAIN FREE life. He sold my husband but hey, it's my body that will be disjointed; I did say pain makes me a Grouch. I had to decide, Dr Patrick or Pain?

Pain will motivate you to step out of your comfort zone. So I finally gave in; besides, I don't think my husband would let me go home without getting help.

So from October 21,2014 until now, Baker Chiropractic and Wellness has reduced or eliminated my pain and numbness, all without medication or surgery!

My shoulder, arm and thumb are back to 90%. Compression on spine, relieved, who knew that stopped migraines. Ribs not right, relieved, restored flexibility helped me with my grandbaby, tying my shoes, brushing my hair, reaching overhead, lots of everyday basic movements.

Chiropractic Adjustments (new word for me) help without hurting and the results are a better life. Adjustments are needed to return your body to its rightful alignment. I have gone to Dr. Patrick Baker, Dr. Joe Fields and Dr. Kelly Duffner to be adjusted, all with good results. It is rare today to like all the doctors in one practice, so I feel blessed.

December 2014 saw my husband coming here for his frozen shoulder which was at 15% flexibility, but now is around 80%.

Soon after talking to Dr. Patrick about how our 3 yr old grandson's doctor and surgeon were leaving his walnut-size lymph nodes alone until he turned 5, our grandson started seeing Dr Kelly Duffner in early 2015. The lymph nodes are now pea size.

Gavin loves going so much that whenever we drive in that direction, he is ready to go. He doesn't understand waiting your turn, so when we arrive, he climbs up on the bed and lays down waiting for Dr. Kelly to FIX him. I tried to explain ADJUSTMENTS to him, but he told me, Dr. Kelly doesn't ADJUST clothes, he FIXES bones. He loves Dr. Kelly and the tickle hammer.

Recently, our skeptical daughter started coming due to numbness in her shoulder and neck pain. Let's just say, she never misses her regular visits to Baker Chiropractic and Wellness.

Family doctors are needful and do well, but for this family it will be after our Chiropractic Care. There are no worries as we know that we'll be directed to our family doctor when needed.

Thank you Baker Chiropractic and Wellness family, (Dr. Patrick, Dr. Joe, Dr. Kelly, Jackie, Danielle and John), for your great care now and for many years ahead.

— **Debbie B.**
— **Tom B.**
— **Gavin (Grandson)**

• • • • •

363

69
Neurocardiogenic Syncope

I first came to Doc because of continual back pain. At my consultation I mentioned that I have a condition the doctors have labeled neurocardiogenic syncope, which causes me to faint frequently. I had never met anyone

who had experience with this until Doc informed me that he has handled patients with this: he was sure he could help. I can't say that I believed him right away, but that has changed!

One Sunday I had two episodes and continued to suffer from vertigo and pain into Monday. I went to Doc's that afternoon and in just one adjustment my dizziness subsided! He sent me for a massage, where his staff eased a lot of the pain and the headache. I was amazed and so thankful!

— S. Dickman

70
Osteoporosis

I am 81 years old and had a lot of constant pain. The tests and x-rays showed osteoporosis, scoliosis and osteoarthritis. My medical doctor told me all this caused high blood pressure and prescribed a blood pressure pill.

I began to get completely bent over and had to walk sideways. I would visit the YMCA two or three times per week and exercise in the pool which would help loosen me up.

My daughter made an appointment for me at Baker Chiropractic. My first visit showed my x-ray was a "mess". I am now showing improvements and have faith in this health care practice. I can drive and I can live on my own. Without these caring and dedicated people, I would be in a nursing home. God Bless them!

— A. Gillespie

• • • • •

71
Pinched Nerve

I came to Baker Chiropractic and Wellness in August with pinched nerves, low back pain, sciatica, neck pain, and fibromyalgia. These problems had been going on for 4 to 5 months and prevented me from doing yoga, exercising and living my everyday life.

Prior to coming here, I had been taking over-the-counter medications to treat my symptoms but found no relief.

The chiropractic care I receive at Baker Chiropractic and Wellness is essential for me. It has relieved my pain and increased my mobility, all without having to use over-the-counter or prescription medications.

If not for Baker Chiropractic and Wellness, I would be in a lot of pain today. I definitely recommend this to anyone. The results

I have seen are very promising!

– Nita P.

• • • • •

Rich Pohana suffered from a severe pinched nerve in his back causing back pain, psoas pain and calf pain. After undergoing corrective chiropractic care, he was able to go on and complete the "Death Valley" bike ride and hike.

Rich rode his bike 148 miles, a ride up 13,403 ft of vertical elevation and hiked on foot 11 miles which took him up another 6,140 feet of vertical elevation. Rich stood on top of the mountain and proudly held his Baker Chiropractic Shirt high!

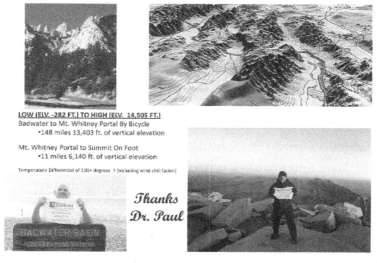

LOW (ELV. -282 FT.) TO HIGH (ELV. 14,505 FT.)
Badwater to Mt. Whitney Portal By Bicycle
•148 miles 13,403 ft. of vertical elevation

Mt. Whitney Portal to Summit On Foot
•11 miles 6,140 ft. of vertical elevation

Temperature Differential of 100+ degrees F (including wind chill factor)

Thanks Dr. Paul

My name is Mary Ann and I am a patient of Dr. Patrick Baker. I have been with Dr. Patrick since August of 2014.

I first came to Baker Chiropractic and Wellness to seek relief from chronic pain in the lower back and lower extremities. I had been experiencing pain, tingling, and numbness for several years and finally

I decided it was time to seek help.

From the very first phone call to his office, up until today, I have been treated as if I were their only patient. Dr. Patrick and his capable staff are consummate professionals and have been such help to me. My initial consultation revealed that I had a pinched nerves and subluxations in the lower lumbar spine. A treatment plan was developed based on my x-rays.

I must admit, I never really knew anything about chiropractic care and was somewhat skeptical. Boy was I wrong! I feel so much better in all areas of my body. What I learned was that not only could Dr. Patrick help my low back pain, but he could also help me with my neck pain, despite the fact that I had a neck fusion surgery ten years ago.

I was always under the misunderstanding that since my neck was fused, I could never be treated by a chiropractor. Lo and behold, I can and my neck hasn't felt this great in years! I owe it to Dr. Baker and his team of knowledgeable professionals.

Dr. Patrick also treats my hands for carpel tunnel and my toes for hammertoe problems. Who knew?!? Fingers and toes as well.

The best part of it all is that Dr. Patrick, all of the other doctors, and the whole healing team really cares about you and your recover. They teach you complete wellness and encourage healthy lifestyles. The entire atmosphere during your visit is very positive and rewarding!

— Mary Y.

72
Professional Athletes Who are Patients

I played with a left hamstring injury since playing college football at Washington University. I went to doctors all over the country to find out what was wrong, and none of the doctors could figure out the problem in my hamstring. I went to Drs. Baker and they found a huge knot in my hamstring and they were able to release it and fix my hamstring problem that I have had since college. I now get adjusted before and after every game. I have been injury free for the past 3 years and have been to the last three Pro Bowls.

— **Corey D, NFL Pro Bowl Running Back**

Playing in the NFL is very physically demanding on my lower

back. Over the last two years of getting adjusted by the Bakers, my lower back has felt 100% better. My lower back is more flexible and strong. I've been injury free since I have been getting adjusted.

— **Brian S.**
Cincinnati Bengals Linebacker

• • • • •

I have never felt better since getting my back adjusted and getting my hamstrings released before and after each game. Since I have been under regular Chiropractic care with Drs. Baker I have been more resilient to injuries and much more flexible. Getting adjusted before and after each game has made a huge difference in my performance

— **Adrian R, NFL Linebacker**

• • • • •

I have been a professional bodybuilder for over ten years and I have literally injured almost every joint and muscle in my body. I have been getting adjusted and massaged at Baker Family Chiropractic regularly for the past two years and I can't tell you what a difference it has made in my life. My neck, shoulders and back feel so much better after getting adjusted. I am able to train with as much intensity now as I did when I was 25 years old. Thanks for all your help Doctors.

— **Franco S.**
IFBB Professional Body Builder

73
Restless Leg Syndrome (RLS)

I grew up with my mom having the occasional back problems from a car accident in her youth. She would get treatment from a chiropractor and the only results that I ever recall observing was my mom tapping the refrigerator magnets along her spine because the chiropractor told her magnets will help heal and put "things" back in place. So, my early impression was you go to a chiropractor only for back problems and magnets was the extent of the treatment. Little did I know...

In the fall of 2016, my mom fell down the stairs and she unknowingly injured her shoulder and neck when she held onto the banister to catch herself. Within a few months of her fall, she could barely lift her arm. Her doctor referred her to see a chiropractor. My mom did her research and she found the *"Best of the Best"* chiropractor in Cincinnati to make sure she got the best possible care. The chiropractor she found was Baker Chiropractic and Wellness on Red Bank Road.

Over the Christmas Holiday, the whole family got together to talk about how we all are and what is new, etc. During this conversation, I was giving my sister-in-law a neck and shoulder massage to work out several huge tension knots that were causing her severe pain and discomfort. Of course my mom, being the wonderful nurturer that she is, wanted to help. She shared her story with us and the progress she made at Baker Chiropractic and Wellness.

Mom told my sister-in-law that Baker Chiropractic was having this amazing holiday special. $21 to get your assessment, x-rays and your first adjustment and encouraged my sister-in-law to make an appointment for the next morning.

My sister-in-law has always had back issues. She broke her back playing competitive soccer in high school and has had sciatic issues ever since. My brother threw his back out about six months prior and still had some residual pain. So, my sister-in-law and brother went to Baker Chiropractic and Wellness the next morning, both taking advantage of the special, and came back with glowing reviews.

My sister-in-law told us how our neck is supposed to be at a 43 degree curve and that her neck was in the negatives. I immediately thought, well if her number is that bad, I know I had to be much worse, since I have horrible posture and the start of a bump on my back. My sister-in-law then showed us this diagram that lists all the things the spine affects. We start going thru the list and all our minds were blown. It was like going thru a checklist of all our aches, pains and random ailments. Therefore, with a combination of my mom, my sister-in-law and my brother saying it was worth it, my sister and I made our appointments.

I have had back pain since my junior year of high school. I was at swim practice one day and suddenly I had shooting pain up and down my spine. I went to the emergency room to see what was wrong. They did several tests and x-rays but they couldn't find anything wrong. I was told since there is nothing wrong, go home, take some ibuprofen and put some ice on it. My back was never the same. I would go through periods of it being fine and just be a dull ache, but then I would bend down, lean too far, pick-up something too heavy, sleep weird, whatever and Bing, there is the shooting pain again. I never would know what would trigger it. I would avoid anything I thought would cause it flair up especially when the ache escalated to a twinge. I knew it was agitated then and I had I to be careful.

Some of my other ailments was that I had been experiencing mysterious nerve issues in my hands. I would have random numbness in my pinky and ring fingers. They would also lock up for no apparent reason. I also suffered from self-diagnosed restless leg syndrome in my left leg. I even had unexplained tummy issues. When I would eat something, sometimes it would be fine, and then sometimes it wouldn't. I had also lost my sense of smell.

January 4, 2017 was my first appointment. It fit in quite nicely with my new year's resolution to actually start going to see doctors and get healthy. My appointment was with Dr. Todd Worthington and he was great. He really explained everything to me in detail. He not only answered all of my questions, but he answered them in layman's terms.

I was shocked to find out how messed up my back truly was. I had subluxations in 5 areas of my spine, hitting 4 of the 5 plexus and the cranial nerves. Basically, my entire nervous system was being affected. My neck was at -3 degrees instead of the 43 degrees, my lower back was over curved, my hips were uneven causing scoliosis in several places, making my spine look like it zig zags, plus disc deterioration in multiple places.

So needless to say, I was a hot mess and I had no clue. I was a little overwhelmed but Dr. Todd was very encouraging saying all of this was reversible, it wasn't some kind of final sentencing. He said with a lot of hard work and commitment, we can turn things around.

We hit the ground running with my treatment plan, I went 3 times week for 3 months. With the combination of the therapy, adjustments and the home kit, I got better. The body is a wonderful thing, it autocorrects as much as possible. But that can be a bad thing too because it is hard to tell when things are wrong. I had no idea I was so off, because feeling off was the norm for me. But once I started to get aligned and my body was being put back together correctly, I felt amazing. I have never felt so healthy and strong. I would call my normal everyday feeling was blah and sickly and I had no idea that is how I was really feeling. I thought it was fine and good. But now thanks to Dr. Todd and Baker Chiropractic I know better. I know what it feels like to really feel good.

My numbers have improved, I am now at 5 degrees on my neck, my hips have leveled out so I am not so zig zaggy, and my posture has improved, I haven't had a back flare up since my treatment started, I am down to the very dull ache and the occasional twinge if I push myself to far. I didn't get sick like I do every winter, my sense of smell has improved and I just feel healthy, like the way my body was designed to feel.

My treatment isn't finished; I still have a long way to go before I am 100%. I have had my own challenges with bump on my back and that will take time to reverse. This is in conjunction with getting my neck to 43 degrees. It has been hindered due to in my second month of treatment, I had my own tumble down a set of stairs and injured my shoulder and neck too. But I was fortunate that I had an appointment the next morning to immediately start work on my shoulder and neck. If I hadn't been going to a chiropractor, I would have ended up similar to my mom and not being able to lift my arm. So, I did a few steps back, but I never lost the momentum forward and I will continue to do so.

This has been a whole family affair for us and we are so grateful to everyone at Baker Chiropractic and Wellness who have help all of us on our journey. We are a healthier and happier family because of their knowledgeable expertise. I would recommend them to everyone.

You never know how much better things could be unless you try!

— **Katrina A.**

• • • • •

I started coming to Baker Chiropractic in October of 2013.

I had trouble with my hands - numbness (but not going totally numb) and tingling about three years ago. My family doctor said it was probably Carpel Tunnel since I was not a diabetic. I just took it for that because it only happened at night and not all the time. Then last year in January of 2013 my feet and legs started with the same tingling, numbness, burning...mostly at night.

I started reading up on the causes of Neuropathy. Oh my gosh, I thought I was going to have something really bad wrong with me. I made another appointment with my family doctor and he told me to go see a neurologist, which I did.

They did testing on me finding out that I did not have Carpel Tunnel or nerve damage in my hands, legs or feet. So he said that I might have Restless Leg Syndrome (RLS) and gave me a prescription for a medication that helps people with RLS. He said he didn't know what was wrong with my hands and that I could get RLS in my hands. REALLY?! So I started on the medication. I also started doing all kinds of research on what causes Restless Leg Syndrome and neuropathy along with all the different things I could do to help it get better.

I TRIED EVERYTHING. I started taking more vitamins. Doctor also said I might have a vitamin B-6 or B-12 deficiency, so I started taking those along with my fish oil and my cholesterol medication (low dose). After about three to four months there was no difference in the way I was feeling.

I now had the tingling, numbness and burning all through the day. I was desperate and thought I was going to have to live like this for the rest of my life. So back to the research. One of my daughter-in laws suggested I should try a chiropractor. I thought what the heck. I've tried everything else, but like others was skeptical about a chiropractor.

I started looking for chiropractors close to where I worked so I could go during the day. I was looking at different websites and found Baker Chiropractic and Wellness. I got on their website, got their number and called. I talked to Danielle and she said "Oh yes we can help" and made me an appointment.

Still skeptical, I went to my first appointment. They did x-rays of my back and neck. Then, I had a consultation with Dr. Baker. Boy was I a mess.....worse than what I could have ever imagined.

He said, "Harvy I can help you, it took you a long time to get this way and it will take awhile to get things back in place". I had pinched nerves in my upper back that caused tingling in my hands. My back was really bad and he said that was the problem with my feet and hands. It all had to do with my nerves!

My husband and I went to the presentation that he gives all new patients and he explained how everything is connected to your spinal cord and nerves and what everything does. WOW, what an eye opener!

Well, I started my first appointment (adjustment) the next week. Dr. Baker had wanted me to come three times a week to start, but I could only come two days a week. By my third adjustment, the tingling and numbness in my hands was almost gone. Now they hardly bother me. AWESOME!

Everyone at Baker Chiropractic is so nice and helpful, they are wonderful.

Both Dr. Patrick and Dr. Paul are always asking how you are doing and REALLY care about you and what you are feeling. You can really tell they care and will try to do everything to make things better. They listen and take the time to answer your questions or concerns and offer suggestions on things to do. They encourage you and explain why this or that might be happening.

My legs and feet are much better than before. There are some days (several days) when they don't bother me at all. I still have my days with the left side of my leg and feet, BUT NOTHING LIKE BEFORE. .AWESOME!

THEY DEFINITELY HAVE A GIFT FROM GOD... Healing in their hands.

THANK YOU SO MUCH Dr. Patrick, Dr. Paul and everyone at Baker Chiropractic and Wellness for helping me feel better again.

— **Harvy T.**

· · · · ·

74
Rotator Cuff

On January 31st, I had a hard fall on the ice directly on my left shoulder. I thought I broke my shoulder, so I had it x-rayed the next morning. It was not broken but there was damage to the rotator cuff.

I had terrible pain trying to move my arm up and down and out to my side. The worst pain was trying to put my arm in my sleeve while putting on a shirt or jacket. This pain didn't get any better after 2 months so I was very concerned that surgery would be required to fix it.

My friend Evelyn was convinced Dr. Paul Baker could help me but I did not think a chiropractor could fix a rotator cuff but I thought I would give him a chance.

After the first 10 visits, I had no noticeable improvement. Dr. Paul said it would get better so I stayed with it. After 36 visits and 20 massage therapy treatments, I'm now healed. I have full motion of my arm and saved myself from surgery.

Dr. Paul Baker did most of my treatments but Dr. Joe Fields also adjusted me. Thanks to these two guys, they got me back to normal. They have been a real blessing to me and I also cannot forget the staff for their care in fixing me.

Dr. Paul has a great staff that remember your name when you come in and are quick to get you on the therapeutic machines. They don't waste your time.

I would be quick to recommend Baker Chiropractic and Wellness to my friends so they can get the best professional chiropractic adjustments.

– John W.

· · · · ·

For some time I have been suffering from a rotator cuff problem with my left shoulder. It finally became so debilitating that I went to orthopedic surgeons who took x-rays and an MRI. One of the surgeons recommended arthroscopic surgery.

Instead of doing that, I started physical therapy, which helped a bit, but I still had a major problem. The problem continued to worsen, and I went to a chiropractor. This also did not work and my shoulder became much worse. It was so bad that I could no longer exercise, my range of motion was severely limited and getting worse, I was unable to sleep on my shoulder, and it was waking me up every night and causing me to be very tired because of the disruption of sleep. And my shoulder was in constant pain.

Then I saw Dr. Patrick Baker when I was walking my dogs, and he asked how I was doing. When I told him of the above, he asked me to give him two weeks for a total of 6 visits. I was at this point highly skeptical and told him so. But I had nothing to lose. So I went to see Dr. Patrick at his office in West Chester, Ohio.

What Dr. Patrick accomplished in just two weeks was nothing short of miraculous to me. I am a lawyer and not prone to exaggeration or impressed easily, and I do not tell people something that is not true. I am incredibly impressed with what Dr. Patrick has done for me.

My range of motion is almost completely restored in my shoulder. I no longer have active pain. I can sleep on my shoulder, and I am again able to exercise with it. It is not yet perfect, but the improvement is dramatic. I would not have believed what he has done for me except that I have experienced it first hand. He has made a huge difference in my well-being and the quality of my life.

Thank you Dr. Patrick.

— **Tom G.**

• • • • •

75
Sciatica Pain

I grew up with my mom having the occasional back problems from a car accident in her youth. She would get treatment from a chiropractor and the only results that I ever recall observing was my mom tapping the refrigerator

magnets along her spine because the chiropractor told her magnets will help heal and put "things" back in place. So, my early impression was you go to a chiropractor only for back problems and magnets was the extent of the treatment. Little did I know...

In the fall of 2016, my mom fell down the stairs and she unknowingly injured her shoulder and neck when she held onto the banister to catch herself. Within a few months of her fall, she could barely lift her arm. Her doctor referred her to see a chiropractor. My mom did her research and she found the **"Best of** *the Best"* chiropractor in Cincinnati to make sure she got the best possible care. The chiropractor she found was Baker Chiropractic and Wellness on Red Bank Road.

Over the Christmas Holiday, the whole family got together to talk about how we all are and what is new, etc. During this conversation, I was giving my sister-in-law a neck and shoulder massage to work out several huge tension knots that were causing her severe pain and discomfort. Of course my mom, being the wonderful nurturer that she is, wanted to help. She shared her story with us and the progress she made at Baker Chiropractic and Wellness.

Mom told my sister-in-law that Baker Chiropractic was having this amazing holiday special. $21 to get your assessment, x-rays and your first adjustment and encouraged my sister-in-law to make an appointment for the next morning.

My sister-in-law has always had back issues. She broke her back playing competitive soccer in high school and has had sciatic issues ever since. My brother threw his back out about six months prior and still had some residual pain. So, my sister-in-law and brother went to Baker Chiropractic and Wellness the next morning, both taking advantage of the special, and came back with glowing reviews.

My sister-in-law told us how our neck is supposed to be at a 43 degree curve and that her neck was in the negatives. I immediately thought, well if her number is that bad, I know I had to be much worse, since I have horrible posture and the start of a bump on my back. My sister-in-law then showed us this diagram that lists all the things the spine affects. We start going thru the list and all our minds were blown. It was like going thru a checklist of all our aches, pains and random ailments. Therefore, with a combination of my mom, my sister-in-law and my brother saying it was worth it, my sister and I made our appointments.

I have had back pain since my junior year of high school. I was at swim practice one day and suddenly I had shooting pain up and down my spine. I went to the emergency room to see what was wrong. They did several tests and x-rays but they couldn't find anything wrong. I was told since there is nothing wrong, go home, take some ibuprofen and put some ice on it. My back was never the same. I would go through periods of it being fine and just be a dull ache, but then I would bend down, lean too far, pick-up something too heavy, sleep weird, whatever and Bing, there is the shooting pain again. I never would know what would trigger it. I would avoid anything I thought would cause it flair up especially when the ache escalated to a twinge. I knew it was agitated then and I had I to be careful.

Some of my other ailments was that I had been experiencing mysterious nerve issues in my hands. I would have random numbness in my pinky and ring fingers. They would also lock up for no apparent reason. I also suffered from self-diagnosed restless leg syndrome in my left leg. I even had unexplained tummy issues. When I would eat something, sometimes it would be fine, and then sometimes it wouldn't. I had also lost my sense of smell.

January 4, 2017 was my first appointment. It fit in quite nicely with my new year's resolution to actually start going to see doctors and get healthy. My appointment was with Dr. Todd Worthington and he was great. He really explained everything to me in detail. He not only answered all of my questions, but he answered them in layman's terms.

I was shocked to find out how messed up my back truly was. I had subluxations in 5 areas of my spine, hitting 4 of the 5 plexus and the cranial nerves. Basically, my entire nervous system was being affected. My neck was at -3 degrees instead of the 43 degrees, my lower back was over curved, my hips were uneven causing scoliosis in several places, making my spine look like it zig zags, plus disc deterioration in multiple places.

So needless to say, I was a hot mess and I had no clue. I was a little overwhelmed but Dr. Todd was very encouraging saying all of this was reversible, it wasn't some kind of final sentencing. He said with a lot of hard work and commitment, we can turn things around.

We hit the ground running with my treatment plan, I went 3 times week for 3 months. With the combination of the therapy, adjustments and the home kit, I got better. The body is a wonderful thing, it autocorrects as much as possible. But that can be a bad thing too because it is hard to tell when things are wrong. I had no idea I was so off, because feeling off was the norm for me. But once I started to get aligned and my body was being put back together correctly, I felt amazing. I have never felt so healthy and strong. I would call my normal everyday feeling was blah and sickly and I had no idea that is how I was really feeling. I thought it was fine and good. But now thanks to Dr. Todd and Baker Chiropractic I know better. I know what it feels like to really feel good.

My numbers have improved, I am now at 5 degrees on my neck, my hips have leveled out so I am not so zig zaggy, and my posture has improved, I haven't had a back flare up since my treatment started, I am down to the very dull ache and the occasional twinge if I push myself to far. I didn't get sick like I do every winter, my sense of smell has improved and I just feel healthy, like the way my body was designed to feel.

My treatment isn't finished; I still have a long way to go before I am 100%. I have had my own challenges with bump on my back and that will take time to reverse. This is in conjunction with getting my neck to 43 degrees. It has been hindered due to in my second month of treatment, I had my own tumble down a set of stairs and injured my shoulder and neck too. But I was fortunate that I had an appointment the next morning to immediately start work on my shoulder and neck. If I hadn't been going to a chiropractor, I would have ended up similar to my mom and not being able to lift my arm. So, I did a few steps back, but I never lost the momentum forward and I will continue to do so.

This has been a whole family affair for us and we are so grateful to everyone at Baker Chiropractic and Wellness who have help all of us on our journey. We are a healthier and happier family because of their knowledgeable expertise. I would recommend them to everyone.

You never know how much better things could be unless you try!

— **Katrina A.**

• • • • •

In June of 2005, I injured my back, severe enough for me to be issued a handicapped parking sticker. The injury to my sciatic nerve inhibited my ability to walk.

Through chiropractic care from Dr. Todd Worthington and implementing a nutrition program, I was able to get completely off my pain medication, Vicodin, within 30 days.

At the time of my injury, I was an obese couch potato and had the profile of Santa Claus. I am now 70 pounds lighter than I was 12 years ago.

Having lost the weight and being pain free, I was able to begin jogging, then running, and then sprinting. I am now participating in Senior Olympics and Master's competition as a track sprinter.

Today, I am 66 years old competing in the 65-69 age group (Medicare bunch) and training with junior high and high school kids.

I am blessed to be rated both nationally and internationally. In 2011, I was the 5th fastest in the 100M at the World Masters competition and 7th in the 200M. I have also earned approximately 20 All-American honors from USATF (United States of America Track & Field) over the last 7 years.

In October 2016, my sciatic issue returned due to arthritis and scoliosis on two areas of my spine. Through treatments from Dr Todd Worthington at Baker Chiropractic and Wellness, all sciatic nerve pain has again been resolved.

Most recently in May 2017, my lower back was strained one week before the 2017 National Senior Games due to my intensive training. Dr. Todd Worthington made almost daily treatments before the competition which allowed me to successfully compete. I was 5th in the nation in my age bracket (65-69) in the 400m, which also earned me an All-American honor. Also I won a gold medal in the 4x100M relay and set a new national meet record.

With my chiropractic care from Dr. Todd Worthington at Baker Chiropractic and Wellness along with my nutrition program, I have gone from a handicapped sticker to winning 6 national championships (gold medals) in track competition and I have transformed myself from being "Fat Freddy" to "Fast Freddy!"

— **Freddy W.**

• • • • •

Dr. Paul Baker has enabled me to walk again without pain and without limping.

I developed severe pain with sciatica in my right leg at age 56. The MRI showed 2 herniated discs. Being a nurse anesthetist, many of the nurses and physicians I worked with who had back problems and opted for surgery, some having 2 or 3 back surgeries, resulted in continued back problems. Therefore, I decided back surgery was not for me. I would just live with the pain.

At age 60, I joined BEAT Training and my trainer recommended Dr. Paul. I was very skeptical, but I decided to see if chiropractic treatment would help relieve my sciatic pain. I was completely amazed when my sciatic pain was cured.

Then I made a big mistake, I stopped going to therapy once the pain was gone. At age 64, I developed arthritis in my right knee with severe leg pain. My x-rays showed both meniscus torn so I had arthroscopy but continued with leg pain and limping. After suffering for another year, I came back to Dr. Paul Baker. Again, with chiropractic treatment, my leg pain and limp were cured.

I have learned that chiropractic care is necessary for one's neuromuscular well-being. I will never again stop receiving chiropractic care and I want to thank Dr. Paul for returning me to a normal and active lifestyle.

— Jessica S.

• • • • •

I came to Baker Chiropractic and Wellness in August with pinched nerves, low back pain, sciatica, neck pain, and fibromyalgia. These problems had been going on for 4 to 5 months and prevented me from doing yoga, exercising and living my everyday life.

Prior to coming here, I had been taking over-the-counter medications to treat my symptoms but found no relief.

The chiropractic care I receive at Baker Chiropractic and Wellness is essential for me. It has relieved my pain and increased my mobility, all without having to use over-the-counter or prescription medications.

If not for Baker Chiropractic and Wellness, I would be in a lot of pain today. I definitely recommend this to anyone. The results I have seen are very promising!

— Nita P.

• • • • •

I would not be in the physical condition I am today without chiropractic care.

I came to Baker Chiropractic and Wellness on June 16, 2016 with pain in my lower right back and sciatic nerve. For more than 3 days, I had been in the worst pain I have ever encountered. I was totally incapacitated.

I attempted to relieve the pain with pills but had zero results. My wife and others suggested I look into chiropractic care for relief. So my wife set me up with an appointment at Baker Chiropractic and Wellness ASAP.

After only two (2) visits, I got relief from the pain! Chiropractic is the only way to go. This was the greatest decision I ever made to care for my body and mind.

I would and do recommend chiropractic care to everyone I encounter who is experiencing a health problem of any kind. You can have anyone contact me for a recommendation, it's for real!

Baker Chiropractic and Wellness is "The Place" for physical and mental betterment.

— Ron L.

• • • • •

I was bound to a wheel chair and a walker since March of last year. I couldn't walk or put any weight on my right leg. When I tried it would just give out. My leg just wouldn't support my weight. I couldn't even drive my car because my right leg wouldn't work well enough to push the gas pedal and the brake.

The pain in my back and leg was so bad I would rate it a 10 on a scale of 1 to 10.

I had been to 5 medical doctors: Different orthopedics doctors who both said they couldn't help me; my regular medical doctor who said I had to live with it; and my oncologist who said, "I just don't know what to do for you." So after 5 doctors said they couldn't help me, I was lost.

Then one day Kathy, a patient of Dr. Patrick Baker, said I had to see him. Kathy told me Dr. Baker has helped many patients with peripheral neuropathy and a pinched sciatic nerve. So I made an appointment and consulted with Dr. Patrick Baker.

Dr. Baker performed an initial examination. A nerve scan showed I had multiple areas of subluxation, and x-rays confirmed it. I was put on a treatment program to correct my subluxations.

To my amazement I went from a wheelchair, to a walker, to a cane and now I do not need anything at all to walk!

The results I have seen are amazing. Just not having to use a cane is unbelievable.

When I first consulted with Dr. Baker I never thought I would ever walk without some kind of walking device.

For the first time since March 2015, I was recently able to drive to Dr. Baker's office myself for my chiropractic adjustment. Before this, I had to rely on someone to bring me to the office. What a relief it is now to be able to drive myself.

Today my pain is virtually gone and I'm improving with every continued chiropractic adjustment.

I can't thank Dr. Patrick Baker and his amazing staff enough. You helped me get my life back!

— Carol L.

• • • • •

I have been seeing Dr. Paul Baker and Dr. Garrett Knuckles for about six months now and I am very happy with the results.

For the past five years I have had extreme pain in my lower back, legs and abdomen areas. I had seen about ten doctors over that period of time in the pain management, orthopedic and other specialists trying to come up with a solution to my problem. This was a very depressing and painful path for myself as well as my family but I was finally brought to Baker Chiropractic and Wellness.

This is the first time I didn't hear surgery or medication was going to be needed. Dr. Paul and Dr. Garrett both spent time with me not just adjusting but talking to me about ways to improve my situation. For the first time I felt like someone took a real interest in my health and was trying to find a solution. I am not 100% yet but I am more than 50% better than I was six months ago.

The best part about my entire experience at Baker Chiropractic and Wellness is the actual staff. They are friendly, caring, and always courteous to my needs.

I will certainly recommend Baker Chiropractic and Wellness to my family and friends. Two thumbs up!

— **Steve C.**

• • • • •

I came to Baker Chiropractic and Wellness on June 11, 2015 with a very severe case of sciatica, lower back pain on my left side, stiff neck and shoulders and dizziness.

My neck and shoulders had been bothering me since December of 2014. My lower back started bothering me in April 2015 and turned into sciatica.

I had visited my personal physician where I was prescribed

anti-inflammatory medication and sent to physical therapy which I felt made my lower back worse.

I had trouble doing my job and taking care of my home.

I saw a commercial one evening where a woman described her symptoms and they were the same as mine. She said that Dr. Baker helped her. That's when I decided to come to Baker Chiropractic and Wellness.

At the present time, I have more mobility in my shoulders, no more dizziness and my back pain and sciatica have lessened.

I feel that I was able to avoid surgery by coming here for chiropractic care.

If you have any problems with your neck, back or hips, I highly recommend checking into chiropractic care and going to Baker Chiropractic and Wellness.

— **Mark Z.**

• • • • •

I first stepped foot into Baker Chiropractic because of severe pain radiating in my neck.

I have suffered from recurring whiplash caused from bus accidents as a child that would flare up three to four times a year. I was used to experiencing the pain. But this last flare up wouldn't go away and practically debilitated me.

Three weeks later, the stabbing and throbbing pains made it difficult to work, stand, sit, and impossible to drive or sleep. Then I met the great people at Baker Chiropractic and Wellness.

Dr. Brock (Frear) took me under his wing and I saw results within a few visits. He took the time to explain his evaluation of my x rays and to show me the subluxations in my spine that were the source of my pain.

In addition to the neck misalignment, Dr. Brock showed me how my hips were also out of alignment. I told him it was probably because I was babying a hurt knee. He replied that my knee was hurting because my hips were offset. He also commented on the fact that he would have thought I had issues with sciatica. My mouth dropped open as I admitted I did have on again/off again sciatic pain.

One adjustment later and I could definitely see a marked difference, not only in my neck but also in my knee. I had more range of motion in my neck, a decrease in pain, I could finally sleep at night, not to mention that I could climb stairs like a normal person again. (side note: I was not at the time suffering from sciatica so I don't know if that was solved or not – but with everything else that improved, I have no doubt that it has as well). After a couple of weeks, I felt like the old me... but better.

It's a joy to go to Baker Chiropractic and Wellness. Not only do I know that I'm correcting my health issues but also the warm and friendly atmosphere is welcoming and makes it a joy to be there. I love the holistic approach and the positivity that radiates the entire practice.

The addition of the massage therapy has helped heal the aches and pains and further preps my muscles and joints to accept the adjustments. And the home therapy gives me the tools to aid me to keep my back healthy.

Dr. Brock and all his staff have a passion for the work they are doing. They each have their own personal story to tell on how chiropractic care, specifically from Baker Chiropractic and Wellness, has enriched their lives and made their health better. It's refreshing to see people love the work they are doing....to the point where Dr. Brock says this isn't work for him and that he sees it as his joy/mission to help all of us live a happier, healthier life.

I, for one, am greatly appreciative.

I'm a true believer in Chiropractic Care from Baker Chiropractic and Wellness. I came to Baker Chiropractic to alleviate my neck pain but also found the cure for my knee and sciatic pain as well, not to mention making my other internal organs healthier. Life can't get better than that!

— Patricia B.

• • • • •

I became a patient of Baker Chiropractic and Wellness by coincidence or I like to think of it as FATE. I was going to watch a TV show that I had recorded but before the show began there was a commercial for Baker Chiropractic and Wellness. On the commercial were two very nice looking & energetic guys talking about what they can do for people suffering from the same things that I was suffering with.

Now I've been to a chiropractor many times in years past so I was no stranger to that type of practice but something about what they were saying intrigued me so I listened further. Their whole delivery sold me & I thought, what the heck, let's give them a call & see what it's all about. On July 2, 2015 I became a patient of Baker Chiropractic and Wellness. It's been three months & I'm here to sing their praises!

I have had chronic sciatica for about twenty years. Within the last few years I became a casual runner, nothing huge, just an occasional 5K for a good charity. This year I upped my game and ran the 10k Flying Pig. Shortly after the Flying Pig I really started to have trouble with my sciatica. It got to the point that when running I could no longer stop & walk when I had to catch my breath.

The pain in my back radiating down my buttocks & leg was so strong that I had to just stop and stand still. I was having difficulty walking up the steps to get into my house due to to the pain and weakness in my back & leg. I tried soaking in a hot tub after my runs but that didn't help. I began taking more over the county anti- inflammatory medicine which in turn started to bother my stomach. I was becoming a mess! That's when I saw the commercial and to this day, I have not seen the commercial since. That's why I call it FATE.

My first day in the Baker Chiropractic and Wellness office was amazing. I had never had a chiropractic practice put me through tests the way they did. I then went into the room where they adjust you and this is when I met Dr. Garrett Knuckles. He was so sweet and kind and gave all indications that he truly cared. He told me that my back was in poor shape and he was so glad I came in. He explained that the disk in my lumbar area was very narrow but the good news was that since there still was some disc to work with they would get me back in shape. I have to admit, I was quite skeptical as it all seemed too good to be true.

I remember walking into the office on my second visit and everyone in the office knew my name. I was totally amazed! With any other doctor that I've gone to for years, no one in the office knew my name until I told them. Yet at Baker Chiropractic and Wellness, when you walk in everyone greets you and asks you how you're doing today.

They're also very accommodating to work with in scheduling appointments. I thoroughly enjoyed the meeting they have with the group of new patients. It is so informative. I can't believe how much I learned and now I'm passing it onto my family and friends.

It's been three months since I first walked into Baker Chiropractic and Wellness and I can't tell you how happy I am with my progress. In three weeks I plan to run my first half marathon and it's all thanks to Dr. Garrett and the staff at Baker Chiropractic and Wellness.

I did have to stop running for a bit, but looking back, that was a small sacrifice for the benefits I am reaping now.

— **Robin F.**

• • • • •

Doctor Paul Baker and his wonderful staff are the best, the most effective, and enjoyable healing experience I've ever had.

The warmth and friendliness of Dr. Paul and his staff have a wonderful healing effect on the stress and tension you feel when you walk into the office and you're in pain.

The main ailment I've been treated for was sciatica (lumbar #5, down the left leg). It was so painful at first, that I had real difficulty just getting out of bed, showering and getting dressed for work.

The first few weeks I received frequent adjustments due to the pain. During those few weeks, the pain became more manageable and fewer adjustments were necessary. Now, thanks to Dr. Paul and his staff, I can comfortably go for weeks between adjustments.

A few months ago, I began to experience slight dizzy spells (vertigo). Some days it was more pronounced, and other days it would fade away. I had no idea that a chiropractor could treat vertigo, and since I dreaded the idea of going to a medical doctor, I felt boxed in with no options. Also, although it didn't affect my job, I was concerned that it might later on. While worrying about this, I casually mentioned it to Dr. Paul one day. Dr. Paul is a very positive and optimistic person, and confident of what he can do with his considerable skill. He smiled and said he could take care of this problem and he did! The procedure took about two minutes! With that one adjustment, about 90% of the problem was gone. I was amazed!

Due to some injuries, I had to visit several chiropractors in the 1970s and 1980s. They were very helpful to me, but I notice that Dr. Paul has a higher level of skill and versatility. I know that he loves his work. I believe that his noticeable determination to give the best service to each patient elevates him to an exceptional level of professionalism.

Another area that exhibits superiority in skill over the 1970s and 1980s are the massage therapists. The knowledge of nerves, muscles and physical technique is noticeably advanced.

Again, the warm and courteous welcome from the nurses, reception, clerical, massage therapists, Dr. Paul Baker and assisting chiropractors genuinely alleviates the emotional tension from any physical pain that we patients may be feeling each time we walk into the office. I would like to say thank you to these caring and attentive workers!

Thank You!

— **Michael S.**

· · · · ·

"I walked into Baker Chiropractic with a sciatic pain attack from a compressed disc. I thought I would never recover. I have never experienced pain like this. The pain was worse than labor pains!

Dr. Paul Baker told me with treatment I would get better. I had a friend that had an attack the same time as I and to date is still in pain and considering surgery.

So back to my story, Dr. Paul gave me my treatment four times a week which included adjustments and massage therapy.

I can tell you that I was unable to sit, stand, walk or lay on my side when I first came to Dr. Paul. Five weeks later, I was doing all of these things.

My nerves calmed down, my inflammation was reduced and all without pain or muscle relaxers. My treatment plan was the key.

I would recommend Dr. Paul, Baker Chiropractic and the entire staff to anyone. Without this group of caring people, I would probably have had an unnecessary surgery at a high expense.

Thank God for Baker Chiropractic!"

— Phyllis H.

• • • • •

Last year, nearing the age of 70 I had three choices: 1. Have a back operation, 2. Use a cane and wheelchair or 3. Live my life on pain pills. Being an active grandmother of four this wasn't on my agenda. Doctors told me there were discs pinching my nerves that were causing sciatica pain to travel down my left leg into my foot.

Excruciating migraine headaches also caused more pain creating the need for pain pills. I decided to try one more thing desperately hoping it would work. After limping into the office of Baker Chiropractic and filling out a medical form, one question being, on a scale of 1-10, ten being severe, what is your level of pain? Mine was 10 and 1/2. After giving me an x-ray and discussing my problems Dr. Paul Baker told me that he could eliminate my pain and I would have no need for pain pills.

Within the first few visits there was definite relief. The exercises, therapy and adjustments caused the migraines to go away first. My leg was a different story though. With each visit Dr. Paul assured me that the pain didn't occur overnight and that he would correct my problem. I have come to find out that as one matures it takes a little longer to heal. Due to Dr. Paul's continued expertise in releasing muscle tightness, knowledge of the body and continuing adjustments my pain level has decreased 95%, which he has told me will be down to 0 very shortly.

Now I can walk 3 miles every day, shop at the mall for 4 hours, dance with my granddaughters (taught them how to jitterbug) and take vacations requiring sitting for long periods of time, without the need of pain pills. Dr. Paul and his staff are very friendly and efficient. I sing their praises to all my friends and truly thank the day I walked into the office of Baker Chiropractic.

— G. McGurrin

• • • • •

My journey at Baker Chiropractic and Wellness began early in 2015 at the recommendation of my daughter. I must admit that I was a bit skeptical.

I came here after having lower back pain that extended down both legs for over ten years. I had been seen by several "top neurologists" who each referred me to the "next best" doctor. I had been treated with decompression surgery and medication therapy.

I saw a neurologist who told me there was nothing more that could be done and I should just continue the medication therapy. I was dependent on a cane. Extensive walking or going up and down stairs was extremely difficult.

I felt I had nothing to lose when my daughter recommended coming to Baker Chiropractic and Wellness.

After several months here, Dr. Paul (Baker) said, "You're walking better". To be honest, I hadn't paid it much attention but now I need the cane much less and traveling up and down steps is much easier!

I recommend chiropractic care to anyone with a similar health condition. Coming to Baker Chiropractic and Wellness has made a big difference.

— Andrea J.

• • • • •

76
Scoliosis

I am a former Division 1 College Baseball player who has been dealing with double curve scoliosis since at least 2010.

One day I woke up and I could not bare the pain I was dealing with any longer. I decided to head into Baker Chiropractic and Wellness to

meet with Dr. Knuckles. Best decision I could have possibly made, so much so that I am disappointed I did not make the decision years earlier.

After only 3 months of adjustments and exercises given to me from Dr. Knuckles, I made major improvements that have led to incredible improvements in my daily living and have me more motivated than ever to continue the process.

By Dr. Paul Baker, Dr. Patrick Baker and Hundreds of Patients

Everyone wants the quick fix for the pain, but unfortunately that is not the case. I was coming in 3 times a week along with doing daily home-care exercises. It was the consistency and desire to make a change that allowed me to make a difference in my well-being.

I cannot stress enough the importance of taking the step down the chiropractic road. The people here at Baker Chiropractic and Wellness are miracle workers and for that, I will always be grateful for them.

— **Curtis O.**

• • • • •

My daughter, Sophia, was diagnosed with early onset scoliosis at the age of 8. Even though the doctor indicated that early onset scoliosis often has the worst prognosis, the only thing he offered was a watch and wait approach. He would reevaluate her spine every 6 months. If and when the curvature reached 25+ degrees, her only options would be to wear a back brace for 23 out of 24 hours per day or have surgery. Although it was only 11 degrees at the time, I agonized over my daughter's future due to the lack of corrective care options presented, in addition to learning of the death of a friend's relative that suffered from severe scoliosis. We anxiously played the watch and wait game for 2 years, feeling happy when there was little change and devastated as the degree of curvature jumped up to 19 degrees at the age of 10. At that appointment, the orthopedist spent less than 5 minutes with us, announcing the degree of curvature and then requesting we come back in 6 months. Only after questioning him (as he began exiting the room) did he indicate that he would begin bracing her back when her curvature went over 20.

Over the course of those two years, when asked if chiropractic care could correct scoliosis or help in any way, 3 different pediatric orthopedists said absolutely not and highly discouraged us from pursuing chiropractic care. "We would be wasting our money" and "chiropractic care could harm our child" were the messages we received. This is ABSOLUTELY FALSE! Under the care of Dr. Patrick Baker, Sophia's scoliosis was reduced to 9 degrees in just 8 weeks. By traditional medical standards, Sophia no longer has scoliosis. We will continue to work with Dr. Baker to eliminate the remaining curvature; however, even if there was no further improvement, Sophia no longer has to worry about bracing or surgery. Traditional orthopedists do not treat a curvature of 9 degrees.

When asked about chiropractic treatment, what traditional healthcare providers should really say is that they are not qualified to respond. Instead of admitting their lack of medical training in chiropractic, they immediately use their medical "expertise" to frighten parents away from the (chiropractic) practitioners that may actually be able to help them. It deeply saddens and disturbs me that many people avoid chiropractors because of the information their traditional doctors provide. Had we not been personally referred to Dr. Patrick, we probably never would have pursued chiropractic treatment for Sophia's scoliosis. Sophia would have endured bracing and possibly unnecessary surgery. Thanks to the care Dr. Patrick has provided, I no longer fear pediatric chiropractic care. I have complete confidence that Dr. Patrick has my family's best interest at heart and will do everything possible to keep my family well.

I want to express my deepest gratitude to Dr. Baker for eliminating Sophia's scoliosis and providing care that promotes wellness. We are clients, not patients, for life. In addition to expressing my gratitude, I hope that my testimonial will encourage parents of children diagnosed with scoliosis to try corrective chiropractic care at Baker Chiropractic. It's the wisest healthcare decision we have ever made for our child.

— Juli G.

· · · · ·

My name is Kristin Betsch and even though I am only eighteen years old, I have been living with chronic back pain most of my life. I had gone to doctor after doctor, and that eventually led to surgeons. I was diagnosed with scoliosis when I was about ten years old and have been monitored ever since. I was told scoliosis does not cause back pain, but there was no other explanation. The last straw was when they referred me to pain management, this was their final solution. But first, I put my foot down. I stood up for myself and said there was no way I would take pain medication the rest of my life. That's when I found Baker Chiropractic. This practice and all of their staff was truly God-send. It was slow going at first, but I never gave up hope. I don't know where I would be or how I would feel today if I hadn't found Doctor Baker. Now, I don't just get my back adjusted, but anything else you can think of, I get adjusted also. I finally physically feel my age! So THANK YOU to all the staff at Baker Chiropractic, you saved my life!

· · · · ·

Hi, my name is Lauren. In 2002, I was diagnosed with scoliosis and a 90 degree spinal curve. It was so bad that traditional medical care was not helping.

In 2011, I went on-line and found Dr. Paul Baker at Baker Chiropractic and Wellness.

Baker Chiropractic's mission is to empower families to take charge of their own health without using drugs, surgeries or other invasive procedures.

I called for an appointment the next day which consisted of a consultation and an exam.

Dr. Paul Baker and his staff were so welcoming and knowledgeable that I knew this was the right place for me.

I have been going to Dr. Paul for 3 years and counting. It's been an amazing experience!

He has helped me with so many things that I had no idea chiropractic care could help with.

In February of this year (2014), I had new x-rays taken and the results were shocking. The curve from my scoliosis was reduced to 50 degrees!

— **Lauren M.**

· · · · ·

My name is Amelia Aiken and I am almost 16 years old. I found out at Baker Chiropractic in February of 2009 that I have scoliosis. Before I found out that I had scoliosis, I also had allergy problems, terrible headaches, and bad migraines. My problems got worse when my little brother started acting up, but since I have been coming to Baker Chiropractic my problems have been getting better.

Dr. Baker is a miracle worker, because I thought my headaches would never go away. I found out that I also have subluxations and forward head posture. I came here first because I had an accident in the 2nd grade and it has been bothering me ever since. Since I started coming here, it has improved a lot and continues to get better every time I come to Dr. Baker. He is probably the best chiropractor anyone will have and should have. Thank you Dr. Baker!

— **Amelia**

· · · · ·

My name is Karen Tribby and I came to Baker Chiropractic because I was having trouble with my back and trouble walking. I have been diagnosed with osteopina; complications from having scoliosis and TMJ in my left upper jawbone.

I went to see Dr. Patrick Baker because I noticed he helped my co-worker, Craig Boykin with his back and walking. Craig has cerebral palsy and he has trouble with his arm being paralyzed and joints that just do not move as they should. I thought if he could help Craig, then maybe I had a chance for help.

I have been to three medical doctors in the past for other medical problems and none helped. It is very frustrating for me because when you have a serious medical problem and you hear the words, "no help", it is hard to keep your faith in doctors and people in general. To add to my problems, I have a ventro-jugular shunt that is in my skull and I was not sure if Dr. Baker had ever heard of or worked with this type of medical procedure. I was born with hydrocephalus and this is why I have the shunt.

When I first met Dr. Patrick Baker and his staff, I noticed that they are very positive people and are committed to helping their patients live normal and healthy lives.

I began my road to a healthier life with Baker Chiropractic in October, 2011. It has been one year now and I have had amazing results with movement returned to my back, legs, neck and shoulders. I did not realize that these areas were being affected by my back. I will continue my road to a healthier life with Baker Chiropractic for years to come. I want to live my elderly years being healthy and very active.

Thank you very much to Dr. Patrick Baker and his staff, may you continue to keep doing what you do and help people live a much healthier lifestyle!

— **Karen T.**

• • • • •

I first came to Baker Chiropractic and Wellness Clinic a little over a year ago at the recommendation of my granddaughter who had benefited from treatment there.

I was experiencing neck pain and back pain along with debilitating problems due to trauma-inducedscoliosis and spinal deterioration.

Even after years of receiving spinal injections and other chiropractic treatment, physical therapy and neuromuscular massages, which gave some relief, I was still experiencing pain,weakness, headaches and limited activity.

With the excellent treatment I've received at Baker Chiropractic's Clinic, I am practically pain free, enjoying long walks and extended road trips, and regained strength and relief from headaches and my range of movement and flexibility has improved.

Dr. Garrett (Knuckles), my attending doctor at the clinic, gets a special "Thank You" from me. Dr. Paul (Baker) and the entire staff there, I offer my sincere appreciation as well.

I have been very blessed by the excellent care, expertise and knowledge of everyone at Baker Chiropractic and Wellness. There is such an encouraging atmosphere and genuine concern for and dedication to the overall health and well being of all their patients.

They have my highest recommendation to anyone needing assistance in this area.

— **Havalyn A.**

· · · · ·

77
Shoulder Surgery

My first visit to Baker Chiropractic was on January 26th, 2015. I had a motorcycle crash in early December of 2014 and shattered my left clavicle, had neck injuries, and the worst concussion I've ever had. I had surgery and after a little more than a month I started to come in for my back and therapy for my neck and shoulder.

The crash was on December 6th, 2014 and I had surgery December 15th, 2014. The only other treatment I had at that point was my orthopedic surgery. The break in my clavicle was such that the pieces weren't connected at all. It made the left side shorter than my right side. The crash happened at a race track in Florida.

So it took a few days to get back up to Columbus and then I luckily got squeezed in for surgery a week later. And because I was like that for about a week and a half, when the plate and screws were put in it stretched the muscles back out. The muscles on my left side were so tight that I went to the emergency room later that same evening as my surgery.

I couldn't eat, walk, shower, get dressed or do anything else by myself for the first month. My boyfriend had to do everything for me. I slowly started to be able to do things with less assistance after that first month. But even then I was still extremely limited. I wasn't even out of my sling for three months after the surgery.

I had never been in so much pain in my entire life. Even with muscle relaxers the muscles in my shoulder and neck were so tight that another chiropractor tried to adjust my neck but all the muscles around that area were "too tight to be adjusted." They told me to come back when I was more healed and wasn't so limited in movement.

When nothing worked with the other chiropractor, I went to Dr. Patrick Baker. He was able to give me gentle adjustments that didn't put me in more pain than I was already in. I never went back to that other chiropractor again. The adjustments and care I get from Baker Chiropractic are the best I have ever received. And thanks to everyone here, I was racing just a couple months after getting out of my sling - about 6 months after my surgery.

The therapy on my shoulder and neck, adjustments, and massages helped me heal, and are still helping me to heal. It also helps me with racing. Racing and all the other activities that are involved in it are very punishing to my body, especially my back. I'm not sure I'd be able to do all that I do without getting chiropractic care.

It's impossible to know where I would be without Baker Chiropractic and Wellness, but I am very glad that I started going when I did. I have already recommended them to my friends.

I tell anyone that I can about the benefits of chiropractic, especially at Baker's. Everyone here helped me through the tough healing process, and continues to help me excel at my sport. I couldn't be more grateful to them for helping me get back to racing and back to my normal life.

— Jessica J.

78
Shoulder Injury

In the spring of 2017, I started a project in my backyard. While working on that project I injured my right shoulder.

At first I didn't think much of it, although I couldn't raise my arm above my shoulder. I thought it was just soreness and getting older catching up to me.

The problem persisted for a few more weeks and became very painful if I moved my shoulder in almost any direction. It was getting worse rather than getting better and I was also having trouble sleeping with this condition. I was stubborn and let it go for a few months, just dealing with the pain. I finally couldn't take it any longer.

After experiencing going through hernia surgery the year before and dealing with my insurance and a high deductible, I decided to try chiropractor care instead of going to see my regular doctor and an orthopedic doctor.

At first I was a little skeptical. After my first couple visits and my examination/evaluation by Dr. Garrett Knuckles, I was still a little skeptical but thought it best to give it a try. Man was I glad I did.

I was given a plan to have 3 adjustments per week for 3 months. After the first couple weeks I made some decent progress and was very happy with how things were going. Dr. Knuckles had told me that shoulders were tricky at the beginning and that it will take a while to see some good progress.

The next couple weeks, honestly and frankly, were not so good. I didn't think I was making any more progress, and at times thought I was going backwards. The range of motion was staying the same and the pain had actually increased a little. Dr. Knuckles could tell I was getting a little irritated and depressed. He reminded me again this is part of the process, it will get better. Well he was right.

The last 3 or 4 weeks of my treatments I have seen steady improvement in range of movement and very little pain. I almost feel back to normal now at the end of my treatments, having almost full range of motion and no pain.

Dr. Garrett Knuckles and the entire staff at Baker Chiropractic and Wellness were very professional and kind, always making every visit a positive experience. I will recommend them to all my friends and family and will definitely be back for regular treatments.

— Tim V.

• • • • •

I would like to thank Dr. Patrick Baker of Baker Chiropractic and Wellness for his expedient and novel treatment of my frozen shoulder.

A frozen shoulder is extremely painful and there is very limited range of motion. This made everyday tasks very difficult and created problems for me at work.

I had 2 episodes of frozen shoulder in the past and in each case the problems lasted over a year and a half. None of the health care specialists I saw were able to offer any relief.

After Dr. Baker's first treatment and a night's sleep I recovered about 60% of the range of motion. After the 3rd treatment in a week's time I had fully recovered my range of motion and had no pain.

I am deeply grateful to Dr. Patrick Baker and strongly recommend his methods for anyone suffering from frozen shoulder.

— **Paul B.**

• • • • •

"When I first met Dr. Patrick Baker it was at AutoZone. I was recently coming off losing a football scholarship due to a shoulder injury. I was pretty down about everything. I had gone through a year of rehab and I still couldn't do push-ups or bench press or anything related to my shoulders.

When I was talking to Doc, I explained that to him. He started telling me there was a possibility that I had pinched nerves and it wasn't allowing everything to heal properly. I was very skeptical but I thought to myself what could it hurt. We set up an appointment and that was the beginning of my healing.

After my first visit, I felt on top of the world. I had more energy. I went home and did my first push up in a year and half. On my following visit, I told Dr. Baker about that. He told me I'm on the road to being maximized. After about a month of regular chiropractic care, I could do around 25 pushups. I was back to bench pressing 135 lbs.

I'm now about 6 months into Dr. Baker's care and I have received another football scholarship. I have a shot at making it to the pros. I firmly believe that if God would have never sent Dr. Baker and the family at Baker Chiropractic, I wouldn't be able to play football again.

So the skepticism for me and chiropractic care has completely been lifted. I would recommend anyone with an injury to give it a go. It's well worth it!"

— **Robert M #84**

79
Sinus Pain

Early one morning, I sent a message to Baker Chiropractic and Wellness. By 4:00 pm that same afternoon I started on my road to recovery.

Over 10 years ago, I began having chronic ear and sinus infections. I have 2 older sisters and they both

began having ear infections around the same age. They both had PE tubes placed and never had issues with ear infections again.

My primary care doctor treated the infections for a while and then recommended that I see an Ear, Nose & Throat specialist. The first ENT told me that adults don't get chronic ear infections. Basically, he totally blew me off. No treatment was provided!

I found another ENT and was taken seriously. Unfortunately, his interventions did not lead to success. He recommended PE tubes and they worked for about 6 months. Even with the tubes, I had 2 additional ear infections. The last ear infection resulted in the tubes being displaced. The ENT allowed my ears to "heal" and started me on an allergy medication. He also recommended that I see an allergist. I began a long road of twice a week allergy injections. The only thing that I received from the allergy injections was that I no longer have a fear of needles!

Next, the ENT recommended sinus surgery for new, more permanent PE tube placement, and to repair to my deviated septum. I would not recommend sinus surgery to anyone! It was extremely painful and took almost a month to recover from.

About a month after surgery, the ENT figured out why I was taking so long to recovery! I developed Methicillin-resistant Staphylococcus aureus (MRSA). My follow up CAT scan showed that the sinus surgery was not successful. Due to the infection, more scar tissue had formed in my nose and sinuses. His recommendation? Let's do the surgery again! I told him that I needed time to consider my options.

About 2 months later, I woke up in excruciating pain. I called my ENT and was informed that he was no longer in practice. I called my PCP and she was able to find me another ENT. The PE tubes, placed two months prior, were no longer in the place. He removed the tubes from the ear canal and told me to see him in 3 months.

My PCP finally decided that I should see a SINUS guy! I was thrilled that I would finally get relief from chronic pain and pressure. I had another CAT scan done. All my hopes were short lived. The ENT looked at my CAT scan and said that "if I was looking for surgery then I came to the wrong doctor." Surgery was the last thing on my mind. But to get relief, I would have gladly had another surgery! The doctor then recommended that I take allegra and a saline spray daily. He assured me that this would relieve all my symptoms!

A year later, he was dead wrong! In this past year alone, I have seen a doctor over 20 times! All visits were for my ears or sinuses. Even after all those visits, I still had chronic sinus pain and pressure. That pressure led to multiple ear infections in the past year.

After too many sleepless nights, I searched and found Baker Chiropractic and Wellness and submitted an appointment request at 4:00 am. I received a response from Danielle by 8:00 am with an appointment that same day. I was impressed from the moment I walked in the door. Everyone was friendly and professional. I got my first adjustment and was amazed that I had some relief. A month later, I have no ear pain! Sinuses are a work in progress but I have 100% faith that they will get better!

My x-rays showed some low back degeneration. I am a nurse and have assumed that back pain was part of the job! I am thrilled to say it is no longer part of the job! Dr. Patrick Baker is heaven sent! He provided me with a thorough understanding of the purpose of chiropractic care and what my x-rays showed. His warm, caring approach is wonderful! I cannot say enough good things about Dr. Baker and the staff at the West Chester, Ohio Chiropractic Clinic!

Their caring and compassion go beyond anything I have ever experienced! I recently experienced a death of a loved one and was overwhelmed by the support I received from Baker Chiropractic. From a thoughtful touch to a sympathy card, Baker Chiropractic went above and beyond to share my loss. I have never had a doctor that knows so much about me and truly cares!

— **Valerie H.**

• • • • •

I started coming to Baker Chiropractic and Wellness a little more than two years ago. I was experiencing pain with head movement of any kind. I had also been having periods of vertigo over the previous few years. After speaking with my regular doctor about the neck pain and if there was a connection between it and the vertigo, I was not satisfied with her solution of taking medications. That is when I decided to give chiropractic care a try. I was nervous about having someone work with my neck, but something needed to be done about the pain.

Treatment started with an exam and X-ray. I was actually listened to as I explained what was happening with my neck. It was so refreshing to talk with someone who cared and understood. The

X-rays showed the curve in my neck was basically non-existent. He promised that chiropractic treatments could help me. Over the past two years, it really has.

The chiropractic adjustments and treatments started bringing relief to my pain right away. These were combined with recommended home exercises which I still do twice a day. Each follow-up X-ray showed improvement in the curvature of my neck. I was experiencing more neck motion with less pain.

Since starting chiropractic care, there have been no new episodes of vertigo. If I am feeling any change in ear pressure, I let them know at adjustment time. It really helps. I used to experience an average of three headaches a month. Since starting treatment, I have only had a few headaches in the last two years.

An unexpected benefit of chiropractic care has been a huge improvement in my allergies. After moving to Ohio 30 years ago, I started having really bad allergies every spring and fall. It was so bad that I had to use a prescription antihistamine like Zyrtek and Flonase nasal spray. Often I would develop a sinus or ear infection as well. The medications were able to stop the allergy symptoms, but they left me feeling tired all the time. I have not had to take a single antihistamine or use nasal spray in the last two years! I would not say my allergies have completely disappeared, but they have decreased to the point where I can actually live without medication except an occasional decongestant. I have not had any sinus or ear infections either. I no longer have to dread months of feeling like I am living in a medicine fog.

The quality of my life has improved so much since coming to Baker Chiropractic. No matter how I am feeling each time I go, I always leave feeling better. I encourage anyone who is suffering to give them a try. I highly recommend them!

— Jean W.

· · · · ·

80
Speech Delay

My son, Baron, was diagnosed with a speech delay at approximately 18 months in age. At this point, his receptive and expressive speech was accessed as that of a 12 month old (approximately 10 words and a lot of babbling).

He was provided services through a children's hospital which included speech as well as occupational therapy. He also received home visits for speech therapy all with on-going assessments and suggestions for us to practice at home. He made slight progress and was approved to begin school at age 3, which was very difficult for me as I am a stay at home/ work from home mom and didn't want to send him to school and away from me at such a young age.

Over the next few months Baron made slight progress although he did become more outgoing due to his social interactions at school. Still there was no significant improvement and he still lagged behind approximately a year (which in pre-school terms is quite a bit).

By Dr. Paul Baker, Dr. Patrick Baker and Hundreds of Patients

One night while tossing and turning over his speech delays, I decided to to research chiropractic options based on an experience I had heard regarding speech improvement from chiropractic adjustments. Through my research, I located Baker Chiropractic and Wellness and was very impressed immediately.

The website provided valuable information, was user friendly (actually allowed me to schedule on-line) and had a wealth of experience in treatments for many areas to include infants and children with issues such as autism.

I scheduled Baron's appointment. He was assessed by Dr. Brock Frear and his therapy/adjustments began. In very little time, I noticed significant improvement.

Within approximately two weeks he no longer snored, something he had been doing from about age one. He also seemed to breathe much better and not so labored during sleep. Next we saw improvement as he progressed from two to three words, to sentences and the ability to express his wants and needs. He went from pointing or saying "eat" to saying, "I'm hungry, I need to eat breakfast." He now tells us if he wants a waffle or cereal, etc. This is wonderful because before this it was trial and error, giving him foods when I thought he should be hungry and seeing which one he would eat.

His expressive and receptive speech has improved at a tremendous speed and his overall vocabulary is too great to count at this point. He still has improvements to make in engaging in conversation but I am sure this too will come.

I have but one regret, honestly...I wish I had known about this three years ago. I would have taken him to Dr. Brock much earlier and avoided many tears, worries and sleepless nights stressing over his lack of speech.

— **Rhonda B.**

81
Spinal Bifida

I am 43 years old. I was born with Spinal Bifida. I have had 42 surgeries. I have been going to the Baker Brothers for 10 years or more. I go at least 2 or 3 times a week and it is the only thing that is keeping me out of a wheel chair. Trust me when it comes to the effectiveness of chiropractic care.

Having so much pain and joints hurt, there are times the pain goes away for a little while and it is a great day for me. I can get something done at home for a little while or go to the store for shopping and bring the groceries in and it takes a day for me to do this. Then there are days I hurt all over and cannot get anything done.

But I know I have an appointment the next day and just getting adjusted gives me a day back and sometimes the next day I feel like a new person for a while like I can do anything because I know I will have another appointment waiting for me and I can make it through another day.

Thanks to the Baker Brothers! I am still wheel chair free at 43 and still going!

— P. Tuttle

· · · · ·

Update to Paula's Story

I recently saw a medical specialist in April with a problem I was having. When the doctor came in, he looked around and asked how I got there.

I know I had a strange look on my face and said I walked in just like everyone does and pointed to the cane I use.

I asked him why he asked me about how I got to his office. The doctor said he has two other patients with my level of Spinal Bifida that are bound to a wheelchair and thought I would be too.

He asked me what I was doing different.

I said two things:

(1). I am a bullhead and won't take no for an answer and

(2). I see Dr. Baker at Baker Chiropractic and Wellness two or three times each week.

He responded by saying whatever you are doing keep it up. Going to a chiropractor must be working. I thanked him.

Second Update To Paul's Story

For the First time eve in my life, my family doctor's office called me at home. He needed to see me for a check-up. My blood pressure meds needed refilled. So I made an appointment. He checked my blood pressure and it was really good. I asked him if we should start taking me off the pills and he said let's not mess with anything right now since everything seems to be working great.

Then I said I had a question for him about the bad kidney I have had since I was born with spinal bifida. I should have lost my kidneys several times but I had a great doctor. So my question to my family doctor was that my Dad wanted to get tested and have me get tested to see if something ever happened to my Dad, I would get his kidneys. My doctor said let me take a look at your records. Then he said I would be able to keep my kidneys for the next 20 years. No transplant should be in my future.

I also told him I see a chiropractor 3 times a week. He said it was helping with my arthritis, ligaments, joints and keeping me loose and mobile while keeping a lot of pain at bay. He said he approved and to keep going to Dr. Patrick.

— **Paula T.**

· · · · ·

82
Stiffness

I started coming to Dr. Baker when I was 16 years old and I just started driving. It was perfect timing for me because I could drive over to Dr. Baker's whenever I needed him vs. waiting on my parents.

I didn't really start going to Dr. Baker's for any sort of reason except that my dad wanted me to go because he said it made him feel so wonderful. He talked our whole family into going and I decided to go one day I would go. I do not really remember why I finally went but I did and I am so glad that I did!

Earlier that year I had suffered a tail bone injury that was probably really bad in medical eyes but I ended up never going to the doctor for it, I also play goalkeeper and do lots of pounding onto my body from running and jumping onto the hard ground.

Over the years this has cause my body to be wracked out of place from just all the different movement I was doing. I never really even realized it and some of my friends said I used to walk really funny but I never really never knew what they meant by that.

In the end, I ended up going to Dr. Baker and receiving my first adjustment. I'll actually never forget my first adjustment because it was so life changing, literally. Dr. Baker had a very hard time adjusting me as first, he said it was because I was soooooo stiff throughout my body.

It felt great at first then I went home and started feeling terrible. I had to go to bed around 7 o'clock or something because I was like I need to chill out after that adjustment. I woke up the next day though and felt amazing. I knew though I still needed a ton of work done on my body because my body had this stiffness to it that was preventing from doing movements and I didn't even know it before.

It probably took a year to six months to where my body wasn't so stiff anymore, after many adjustments a week and massages. After a while my friends said I lost that weird walk I used to have and my playing in soccer increased dramatically. I felt myself actually become more athletic, which I was super happy about because this was the year that colleges started looking at me. I now was able to perform at a higher level in front of these coaches and make my dreams come true.

Dr. Baker also helped me not have TMJ anymore and if I ever jammed up something in the body he would fix it, every single time.

I am very thankful that I met Dr. Baker. He changed my life with my body performance but his clinic is more than just adjustments.

He cares about you and what you want to achieve in life which is why I always enjoy my visits.

I've known him now for 7 years and I think this is a friendship that will last, plus he always hires the best people to work with him. Mostly everyone in the that office has impacted my life in a way, especially Courtney trying to help me edit my essay, but going to Dr. Baker's is about getting the whole package when you go and that is why his family clinic is so special to me.

— Natalie S.

•   •   •   •   •

83
Tachycardia

"I began being treated at Baker Chiropractic and Wellness in the early part of July. My initial complaint was about a small curve that I noticed forming in my upper back.

Once I was in the office I was given a diagram of the spine. In this diagram it showed how the spine is connected to everything in the body. I already knew this, but I never really knew about it in depth. Once given the diagram and speaking with Dr. Paul Baker, I was educated on how the curve in my spine was affecting my body.

Oddly enough I had been having some small troubles with my heart a few months prior to coming to Dr. Baker. I had not mentioned this to anyone in the office. Once Dr. Baker finished explaining to me what his findings were I asked him if the heart problems I had been experiencing could be coming from the curve in my back. His response to me was "absolutely."

By Dr. Paul Baker, Dr. Patrick Baker and Hundreds of Patients

He explained that the spine is attached to everything in the body, and what I probably had going on was a pinched nerve that lead straight to my heart. This made total sense to me because I had already undergone a series of tests that revealed nothing. I was put on medications that I felt I really shouldn't be taking being that the doctor really didn't know what was causing my ailment.

Dr. Baker began my exercises and adjustments immediately. After about 5 visits I have already noticed a change. My heart ailment is not as pronounced anymore. I am able to sleep. I am not as irritable as I had been over the past few months. Going to the chiropractor for this short time has given me faster results than going to the medical doctor for all of those months. I feel like the medication I was given was to treat my symptoms but Dr. Baker is treating and correcting the problem.

I am so glad I made the decision to go to the chiropractor when I did. Dr. Baker is so honest and warm. Once you encounter him you know that he is genuine and that he is determined to help you to the best of his ability. His staff is the same way. By my second visit they all knew me by name. In a place where they see hundreds of patients a day this was impressive.

They have always greeted me by name and with a smile. If I have any questions or concerns I have no problems being helped.

I LOVE Dr. Baker and his staff. They have truly changed my life."

— **Elease N.**

• • • • •

84
Temporomandib-
ular Joint Disorder
TMJ

I started coming to Dr. Baker when I was 16 years old and I just started driving. It was perfect timing for me because I could drive over to Dr. Baker's whenever I needed him vs. waiting on my parents.

I didn't really start going to Dr. Baker's for any sort of reason except that my dad wanted me to go because he said it made him feel so wonderful. He talked our whole family into going and I decided to go one day I would go. I do not really remember

By Dr. Paul Baker, Dr. Patrick Baker and Hundreds of Patients

why I finally went but I did and I am so glad that I did!

Earlier that year I had suffered a tail bone injury that was probably really bad in medical eyes but I ended up never going to the doctor for it, I also play goalkeeper and do lots of pounding onto my body from running and jumping onto the hard ground. Over the years this has cause my body to be wracked out of place from just all the different movement I was doing. I never really even realized it and some of my friends said I used to walk really funny but I never really never knew what they meant by that.

In the end, I ended up going to Dr. Baker and receiving my first adjustment. I'll actually never forget my first adjustment because it was so life changing, literally. Dr. Baker had a very hard time adjusting me as first, he said it was because I was soooooo stiff throughout my body.

It felt great at first then I went home and started feeling terrible. I had to go to bed around 7 o'clock or something because I was like I need to chill out after that adjustment. I woke up the next day though and felt amazing. I knew though I still needed a ton of work done on my body because my body had this stiffness to it that was preventing from doing movements and I didn't even know it before.

It probably took a year to six months to where my body wasn't so stiff anymore, after many adjustments a week and massages. After a while my friends said I lost that weird walk I used to have and my playing in soccer increased dramatically. I felt myself actually become more athletic, which I was super happy about because this was the year that colleges started looking at me. I now was able to perform at a higher level in front of these coaches and make my dreams come true.

Dr. Baker also helped me not have TMJ anymore and if I ever

jammed up something in the body he would fix it, every single time.

I am very thankful that I met Dr. Baker. He changed my life with my body performance but his clinic is more than just adjustments. He cares about you and what you want to achieve in life which is why I always enjoy my visits.

I've known him now for 7 years and I think this is a friendship that will last, plus he always hires the best people to work with him. Mostly everyone in the that office has impacted my life in a way, especially Courtney trying to help me edit my essay, but going to Dr. Baker's is about getting the whole package when you go and that is why his family clinic is so special to me.

— Natalie S.

• • • • •

I don't remember when it started. But it's safe to say that I have had TMJ for a long time... for most of my life.

I had it long before I had a name for it. It was simply that clicky-jaw-thing. And by clicky-jaw-thing, I mean that thing when you yawn or chew or laugh really hard and your jaw pops... loudly. And someone near you says, "What was that?!" And then you say, "Oh... that was my jaw." Not so much topic of conversation and pretty humiliating.

The clicky-jaw-thing stuck around through all of high school and into college before I knew that there was actually a technical term for it. I finally asked the dentist about it and he said that the clicking was caused by a Temporomandibular Joint disorder, or TMJ. Basically, he said that my jaw was out of line. He suggested a night mouth guard because TMJ can sometimes be caused by nighttime teeth grinding and I was a confirmed teeth grinder.

Over the years, I used a mouth guard from the dentist, bought several from different drug stores, and had another made by a different dentist. They made me talk funny and drool more, but none of them magically aligned my jaw.

At this point, over ten years ago, my dentist was out of options that didn't require surgery. I had no intention of getting jaw surgery and at some point in the last decade I had simply resigned myself to the fact that I would be stuck with TMJ for the rest of my life. Unfortunately, this acceptance included frequent headaches, many doses of ibuprofen, and the all too familiar clicky-jaw-thing.

About six months ago we started seeing Dr. Paul. My husband stumbled upon his name (and by stumbled, I mean divine intervention) and went in for an issue he was having with his back and within a few weeks, our daughters and I were also patients. After the back x-rays were taken, the consultation, and the adjustments, I was feeling great, but it didn't even dawn on me to bring up the TMJ. He's a chiropractor, not a dentist... right?

But then I saw him working on a young woman's jaw. And then I heard another young woman tell him how much better her TMJ has been. I nearly cried. I asked Dr. Paul if he worked on TMJ... of course he does! It's been about three months since he started working on my jaw— just a few minutes after each adjustment— and it has already made a remarkable difference!

I used to get headaches every day. Every day. Many of them would start in my jaw and work their way up to my temples. Frequently I would wake up with a searing headache that was lodged primarily in my jaw.

That is a rare occurrence these days. I rarely have headaches and when I do they are slight not severe. My jaw still clicks, but it doesn't send the jolt of pain that it used to. And I have a larger range of motion... which is to say, I can open my mouth wider without the clicking and the hurting.

The pain lifted steadily. It was a release and an overwhelming relief. As I look back, it is baffling that I had accepted that level of discomfort. But when it started to recede and then go away completely, it was like an entirely new life. Having lived with constant pain and to then watch it disappear, I began to realize just how stressful and all-consuming living with that agony had been. The lightness, relief, and joy that come from its lifting are life changing.

Finding Baker Chiropractic, Dr. Paul, and the entire staff has changed the lives of our entire family. We are healthier, happier, and we feel better than ever! Occasionally I imagine how much Advil it would have taken to get through my life with TMJ, or I think about having to endure a painful jaw surgery or wear some contraption on my face every night while I sleep... and each time I send up a silent prayer for Dr. Paul and the path that led us to him.

• • • • •

85
Tremors and Seizures

My son has experienced tremors since birth. They were mild and infrequent until last year. His pediatrician was never able to precisely diagnose his conditions. We went through numerous tests without any conclusions. Before we began treatment at Baker Chiropractic, he had increased his tremor spells to 4-10 times almost daily.

Since we began treatment at Baker Chiropractic, he has had only 2 or 3 tremors and no tremors whatsoever since January.

We were very skeptical at first but now we wish we would have found Dr. Paul and Dr. Patrick earlier.

— T. Lind

· · · · ·

I was having seizures due to a brain tumor and suffering from severe headaches. I was feeling terrible and was beginning to think that I would have to live life around this pain and stop doing the things I love to do because the pain was so intense. At times, it was unbearable.

After coming to Baker Chiropractic, I began to feel better. The many benefits I have experienced personally from chiropractic care are minimal number of seizures. When I do have them, they don't last as long as before. My headaches are almost entirely diminished and my back pain is much better.

In all honesty, I would have to say I feel better health wise than I have felt in years.

— O. Murrell

86
Torticollis

When Brooke was three months old she was diagnosed with torticollis. Torticollis is the tightening of the muscles on one side of the neck causing the baby to look in only one direction. She was referred to start physical therapy right away. During our first visit with the PT, we were told torticollis could also cause a flattening of the skull on one side or the back of the head, known as Plagiocephaly. This looked like the direction we were heading, which would result in Brooke wearing a helmet for six months; 23 hours a day.

When we started physical therapy they said it would take at least eight months to see any real improvement. Mind you, we were dealing with a very uncomfortable, fussy baby which called for many sleepless nights. More importantly, how would this condition affect her development; her motor skills.

Eight months seemed like an eternity. I was so discouraged and felt really helpless. One day I was talking to our home health care nurse about Brooke's condition and how I was feeling. She told me her neighbor's son also had torticollis and was treated by Baker Chiropractic. She said he was much more comfortable and sleeping a lot better and recommended I give them a call.

I was a little skeptical. I had heard so many different opinions of chiropractic care, but at this point was willing to try anything. I can honestly say this is the best thing I could have done for her. After only 10 visits, there is a dramatic improvement in Brooke's condition. She is like a totally different baby. To look at her now you would never know there was ever anything wrong with her. She holds her head straight, looks in either direction, (sleeps thru the night!!!) and is a much much happier baby. Needless to say, I am a much happier mommy!!

I recently took Brooke back to the PT and they themselves were quite impressed with the progress. Turns out, she won't need that helmet after all. To go from facing eight long months of therapy, to results after 10 adjustments is such a relief and truly amazing. I was so afraid we would miss out on the joy of our baby's first year.

I cannot say enough how grateful we are to Dr. Baker and his staff. Everyone there has been so great to work with. They are always so friendly and genuinely happy to see us. As a mother of four little ones walking into a doctor's office, that's not usually the response I get.

Thank you so much for your dedication in helping Brooke. You have given us back those eight months and lifted a great weight off of our family - I just can't thank you enough for that!!

— S. Garrison

· · · · ·

After much speculation and debate, I decided to succumb to the circumstances and pay Dr. Baker a visit. My newborn daughter, Kendall, had severe feeding issues in that she would spit up most of what she ate at every feeding. In the hospital she would gag and gasp for air it was so severe. I was told that she was having these issues because she was born in less than 40 minutes and it was too quick for fluids to leave her system naturally through the birthing process, and that it would soon cease. After nearly one month of this happening I took her to the pediatrician who diagnosed her with severe acid reflux and prescribed Zantac.

Administering this medicine (for the short time in which I did) was the cruelest thing I have done to any of my children. Although it did seem as if it helped slightly with her gagging and the reflux, the medicine itself was so potent that it would burn my eyes upon smelling it. When I (attempted) to give it to her she would gag, hold her breath and spit it right back at me, and her eyes would water also. After only a few doses, I didn't feel like the side effects of the medicine were worth the benefits, and that there had to be a better alternative. It was then that I was recommended to see Doc.

The more I thought about Kendall's upcoming chiropractic experience, I began to think of other concerns I had. She was always holding her head to one side, and never seemed to develop neck muscles and head control as my other children had at her age. I wasn't quite sure if this was a cause for worry, but it was definitely something that I wanted to address. Our initial meeting with Doc was comforting, informative, and assuring. He addressed all of my questions, and assured me that this was my first step toward living a happier, healthier life for Kendall, I, and the rest of my family.

I was informed that Kendall had a case of Torticollis, and that with adjustments I would see great improvement. So I entrusted Dr. Baker, a father of small children himself, with one of my precious gifts from God and put her health and her future in his hands. For her first adjustment my initial nervousness quickly subsided as I witnessed something amazing. He held her softly between his hands and did his work, and as he did so, she smiled at him and cooed softly putting me to ease. She thoroughly enjoyed what she was experiencing and there seemed to be a weight lifted off my shoulders. Later that night Kendall was in great spirits, and seemed to be less fussy that usual. She was also holding her head up slightly better than usual. I initially played this off as coincidence until our return visits with Doc.

The next time we went, I decided to get adjusted – after all, I had chronic back problems from a wreck and my 50lb+ weight gain from all of my pregnancies had not helped! I walked out of his office feeling like a new person. Instead of walking around and living with a constant ache, I felt something that could not be expressed in words – I literally felt nothing. Kendall and I visited Doc on a regular basis and after just a few visits Kendall's acid reflux had seen a tremendous improvement, and she was holding her head upright as if there had never been a problem. But, most importantly for the both of us, she began sleeping for more than three hours in a row!

My other children have also begun reaping the benefits of chiropractic. My youngest son Kayden, who is two, saw Doc for the first time after an accident in which he received several staples in his head. Doc initially adjusted his neck, but after gaining Kayden's comfort and confidence, he adjusted his back as well. On several occasions Kayden has asked for "Doc to fix neck", and we went to see him!! He even knows the routine and sits patiently in his chair, hands in his lap, for his turn, and then runs to the table and positions himself accordingly for his back adjustments. My five-year-old daughter and son both have been adjusted and they too, have asked on several occasions to see Doc when they were not feeling well. My husband is a landscaper and does snow removal and is constantly on his feet, and constantly saying how badly his back feels. After just one visit he felt tremendously better, and will be returning especially with the grueling winter months ahead of him!

There is no stereotypical chiropractic patient. We come from different backgrounds with different prior experiences, different symptoms, and different goals for relief. Everyone can truly benefit from chiropractic, as I have learned over the past few months, especially with my own family. We all have different symptoms and concerns ranging from acid reflux, constipation, head and neck trauma, ADHD, ear infections, and more! And yet, we all unite under one common ground, that being relief we seek from visiting with Dr. Baker. I have suggested to several family members and friends the benefits they too could achieve.

I would never force or insist chiropractic care upon anyone. I would however, ask that anyone and everyone simply try it one time, and let it speak for itself. They too, would be a life-long patient of Baker Chiropractic!

— The Cortright Family

87
Urinary Incontinence

I had been dealing with urinary incontinence and leakage for several years. I lead a very active lifestyle and this was really becoming a problem. My gynecologist referred me to a urogynecologist who put me on medication and had me doing pelvic floor exercises. She wanted to try these methods before considering surgery to fix the problem.

The medication helped almost immediately, but the side affect was an extremely dry mouth. I felt dehydrated all the time.

I was on the medication for about 3 months when I began to see Dr. Patrick for neck and back issues. After several adjustments I noticed my bladder was emptying differently. I did not see how this would relate to chiropractic adjustments, but decided to mention it to Dr. Baker.

I told him about the incontinence issue and he was glad I did. He advised me chiropractic can cure incontinence. Never in a million years would I have thought that! He told me absolutely not to have the surgery.

The excellent massage therapists at Baker Chiropractic also gave me massages to help relax my bladder. The misalignments in my spine and pelvis had caused my bladder not to function properly.

After several weeks I decided to stop taking the medication; as I was feeling more and more dehydrated. I thought the incontinence might worsen, but it did not. The adjustments and massages I am receiving at Baker Chiropractic are definitely helping with this issue. I feel I am about 95% cured. Who would have thought?

I have no intention of seeing the urogynecologist again!

— J. M.

88
Vertigo

I first visited Baker Chiropractic and Wellness about 7 months ago. I suffered with chronic vertigo and neck problems for over a year.

My ENT physician sent me for extensive medical testing. From his recommendation, I attended vestibular therapy at the hospital and began taking medications. These treatments helped very little.

I did some research and decided to try chiropractic care. I was a bit skeptical.

I met Dr. Kelly (Duffner) on my first visit to Baker Chiropractic and Wellness. He took x-rays and explained the problems with my neck and spine. He was very confident that chiropractic treatment would help me.

After two weeks of treatment, I knew my symptoms were diminishing. I first noticed that my neck no longer hurt. Also, my vertigo symptoms were less intense.

My treatment continued, and after a couple of months, I felt quite a bit better. Treatment at Baker Chiropractic and Wellness has allowed me to return to work and I continue to make progress.

Chiropractic care is the only thing that has helped relieve my symptoms. I no longer need medications.

Dr. Kelly Duffner and Dr. Patrick Baker have been great throughout my treatment and I am grateful for their help.

— Jason H.

. . . . .

In late August of 2015 during one of my daily walks I fell down in the street. I experienced balancing problems in early September and became dizzy. This turned into vertigo.

My doctor prescribed medications for vertigo. This medication didn't work at all. Next I was sent to an ear, nose and throat doctor who said I didn't have a problem in those areas either. He sent me to the Center for Balance in which I was taught coping skills so I could walk without falling down.

My husband had to drive me everywhere. Then my husband,

Patrick, came through for me again and saw an ad for Baker Chiropractic and Wellness. I made an appointment there and was lucky to get Dr. Garrett Knuckles as my new chiropractor.

When I first saw him I felt so depressed and wished that I was dead because I couldn't do anything because of the acute vertigo and I felt worthless. However, Dr. Knuckles promised me that he could cure vertigo and I placed my trust in him.

I saw him three times a week at first. By late spring of 2016 my vertigo was gone.

It is now July and I am still free of vertigo and I can drive again and am taking art classes.

Thank you, Dr. Knuckles who is gentle, kind and experienced. He cured me of a debilitating problem.

— **Adele E.**

• • • • •

I started coming to Baker Chiropractic and Wellness a little more than two years ago. I was experiencing pain with head movement of any kind. I had also been having periods of vertigo over the previous few years. After speaking with my regular doctor about the neck pain and if there was a connection between it and the vertigo, I was not satisfied with her solution of taking medications. That is when I decided to give chiropractic care a try. I was nervous about having someone work with my neck, but something needed to be done about the pain.

Treatment started with an exam and X-ray. I was actually listened to as I explained what was happening with my neck. It was so refreshing to talk with someone who cared and understood. The

X-rays showed the curve in my neck was basically non-existent. He promised that chiropractic treatments could help me. Over the past two years, it really has.

The chiropractic adjustments and treatments started bringing relief to my pain right away. These were combined with recommended home exercises which I still do twice a day. Each follow-up X-ray showed improvement in the curvature of my neck. I was experiencing more neck motion with less pain.

Since starting chiropractic care, there have been no new episodes of vertigo. If I am feeling any change in ear pressure, I let them know at adjustment time. It really helps. I used to experience an average of three headaches a month. Since starting treatment, I have only had a few headaches in the last two years.

An unexpected benefit of chiropractic care has been a huge improvement in my allergies. After moving to Ohio 30 years ago, I started having really bad allergies every spring and fall. It was so bad that I had to use a prescription antihistamine like Zyrtek and Flonase nasal spray. Often I would develop a sinus or ear infection as well. The medications were able to stop the allergy symptoms, but they left me feeling tired all the time. I have not had to take a single antihistamine or use nasal spray in the last two years! I would not say my allergies have completely disappeared, but they have decreased to the point where I can actually live without medication except an occasional decongestant. I have not had any sinus or ear infections either. I no longer have to dread months of feeling like I am living in a medicine fog.

The quality of my life has improved so much since coming to Baker Chiropractic. No matter how I am feeling each time I go, I always leave feeling better. I encourage anyone who is suffering to give them a try. I highly recommend them!

— Jean W.

• • • • •

Doctor Paul Baker and his wonderful staff are the best, the most effective, and enjoyable healing experience I've ever had.

The warmth and friendliness of Dr. Paul and his staff have a wonderful healing effect on the stress and tension you feel when you walk into the office and you're in pain.

The main ailment I've been treated for was sciatica (lumbar #5, down the left leg). It was so painful at first, that I had real difficulty just getting out of bed, showering and getting dressed for work.

The first few weeks I received frequent adjustments due to the pain. During those few weeks, the pain became more manageable and fewer adjustments were necessary. Now, thanks to Dr. Paul and his staff, I can comfortably go for weeks between adjustments.

A few months ago, I began to experience slight dizzy spells (vertigo). Some days it was more pronounced, and other days it would fade away. I had no idea that a chiropractor could treat vertigo, and since I dreaded the idea of going to a medical doctor, I felt boxed in with no options. Also, although it didn't affect my job, I was concerned that it might later on. While worrying about this, I casually mentioned it to Dr. Paul one day. Dr. Paul is a very positive and optimistic person, and confident of what he can do with his considerable skill. He smiled and said he could take care of this problem and he did! The procedure took about two minutes! With that one adjustment, about 90% of the problem was gone. I was amazed!

Due to some injuries, I had to visit several chiropractors in the 1970s and 1980s. They were very helpful to me, but I notice that Dr. Paul has a higher level of skill and versatility. I know that he loves his work. I believe that his noticeable determination to give the best service to each patient elevates him to an exceptional level of professionalism.

Another area that exhibits superiority in skill over the 1970s and 1980s are the massage therapists. The knowledge of nerves, muscles and physical technique is noticeably advanced.

Again, the warm and courteous welcome from the nurses, reception, clerical, massage therapists, Dr. Paul Baker and assisting chiropractors genuinely alleviates the emotional tension from any physical pain that we patients may be feeling each time we walk into the office. I would like to say thank you to these caring and attentive workers!

Thank You!
— **Michael S.**

· · · · ·

I have been coming to Dr. Patrick Baker since March. Prior to becoming a patient, I experienced constant and severe pain as well as dizziness. However, those symptoms are no longer an issue!

I used to take muscle relaxers and pain medicine, but since I've been coming to Dr. Baker's office I no longer need them. The constant pain would sometimes keep me awake at night. Now I am sleeping better and without pain. At home, I would leave certain chores go undone because I was unable to do them without having severe pain. That has been changed around since becoming a patient. Now I feel like I am actually accomplishing things at home.

There were many days at work where I would actually pray to get through my shift because the pain was so intense. However, I am no longer having that problem because most of the pain has subsided.

Another issue I had prior to becoming a patient was vertigo. Every time I would turn my head, I felt very dizzy. It became a regular occurrence but after getting adjusted, the dizziness stopped.

The added bonus of being Dr. Baker's patient is that he and his staff are all wonderful! I feel like I have gained a bunch of new friends!

— S. Thomas

89
Weight Loss
& Medication
Reduction

In June of 2005, I injured my back, severe enough for me to be issued a handicapped parking sticker. The injury to my sciatic nerve inhibited my ability to walk.

Through chiropractic care from Dr. Todd Worthington and implementing a nutrition program, I was able to get completely off my pain medication, Vicodin, within 30 days.

At the time of my injury, I was an obese couch potato and had the profile of Santa Claus. I am now 70 pounds lighter than I was 12 years ago.

By Dr. Paul Baker, Dr. Patrick Baker and Hundreds of Patients

Having lost the weight and being pain free, I was able to begin jogging, then running, and then sprinting. I am now participating in Senior Olympics and Master's competition as a track sprinter.

Today, I am 66 years old competing in the 65-69 age group (Medicare bunch) and training with junior high and high school kids.

I am blessed to be rated both nationally and internationally. In 2011, I was the 5th fastest in the 100M at the World Masters competition and 7th in the 200M. I have also earned approximately 20 All-American honors from USATF (United States of America Track & Field) over the last 7 years.

In October 2016, my sciatic issue returned due to arthritis and scoliosis on two areas of my spine. Through treatments from Dr Todd Worthington at Baker Chiropractic and Wellness, all sciatic nerve pain has again been resolved.

Most recently in May 2017, my lower back was strained one week before the 2017 National Senior Games due to my intensive training. Dr. Todd Worthington made almost daily treatments before the competition which allowed me to successfully compete. I was 5th in the nation in my age bracket (65-69) in the 400m, which also earned me an All-American honor. Also I won a gold medal in the 4x100M relay and set a new national meet record.

With my chiropractic care from Dr. Todd Worthington at Baker Chiropractic and Wellness along with my nutrition program, I have gone from a handicapped sticker to winning 6 national championships (gold medals) in track competition and I have transformed myself from being "Fat Freddy" to "Fast Freddy!"

— **Freddy W.**

• • • • •

If it weren't for God leading me to Baker Chiropractic and Wellness, I would still be in pain and hopeless about it. I put my trust in medical doctors, and they could not help me. Much of the time, it felt like the doctors I went to didn't even believe me – passing me off as a hypochondriac – that my symptoms were "all in my head". They only gave me drugs to treat symptoms or gave me unnecessary surgeries for things that could have been helped with chiropractic care.

Although two years ago I was suffering from a long list of ailments, I came to Baker Chiropractic because I had been having debilitating pain in the back of my head and neck. I used to think my health would just get worse with time and I secretly wished I would die young because I didn't want to think about the level of pain I would be in thirty years down the road – I was already in a great deal of pain presently!

Much to my surprise, Dr. Brock Frear told me he could not only help me with my head and neck, but help me with pretty much everything else I was suffering from! Truthfully, I was skeptical at first – I had been disappointed so many times before. But the fact that he simply believed me and sympathized with me made me want to give him a chance to prove his promises.

After many reassurances, hugs, education on healthy lifestyle choices, plenty of adjustments, treatments, and home exercises – I am a new woman! Those headaches are gone, and when they occasionally try to take hold of me again, adjustments make them disappear! I have gone completely off the antidepressants I had taken for years, I have lost over thirty pounds, I no longer need cortisone shots in my knees nor suffer daily knee pain, my digestion is much improved, and currently the doctors are getting rid of my hiatal hernia! Surgeries are my last resort now, and the supplements offered at Baker Chiropractic take the place of drugs (with no side effects and better results).

The doctors at Baker Chiropractic would love to talk with you – or rather HELP you! They know they can – they have proven results! They genuinely care and are passionate about helping people. Many of them have been in dire circumstances themselves before they found how well chiropractic care works. They are like a family – waiting to adopt everyone who comes in with a desire to be physically well and bless those people with a priceless gift – hope for a brighter future. I am forever grateful to be one of those people!

— Laura K.

· · · · ·

My name is Melissa, I live in Fairfield, Ohio and I'm 57 years old.

When I was 6 months old, I contracted German Measles. This developed into encephalitis and I was diagnosed with epilepsy. For many years, the doctors tried to find a medication that controlled my epilepsy. I was told I would always be taking medication for the rest of my life.

Throughout my life, I discovered many different venues that could help me to live my life as well as possible while on medication. All the different medications I had tried throughout the years have had side-effects. Before coming to see Dr. Brock, I was doing my best to live my life as fully as possible while attempting to ameliorate the side-effects the best I could.

Prior to coming to Baker Chiropractic and Wellness, I had seen many other chiropractors for various reasons. Along the way, I picked up a lot of beneficial information. After coming to Baker Chiropractic and talking to Dr. Brock, I realized I had not been connecting the dots. Knowledge is power but power without proper implementation is fruitless.

My primary care physician had NEVER told me reduction or elimination of my medication was possible. The doctor was more than happy to keep refilling my medication month after month, year after year. I have an upcoming appointment and I look forward to the doctor's reaction! This is MY DREAM- being TOTALLY OFF my epilepsy medication PERMANENTLY!!

After only 23 visits to Baker Chiropractic, approximately 2 1/2 months (not EVEN 90 days!), I was 100% free of ALL my medication! Before talking to Dr. Brock, I had not been given any hope of EVER being off my medication.

Prior to coming here, I had been able to reduce my medication through vitamin and mineral supplementation but ELIMINATING all medication, did not seem to be a possibility. I can't tell you the number of times I have agonized over my level of care in my elderly years. "Who is going to make sure I get my medication every day?" I did not want to be a burden to anyone. I have always tried to live as healthy a lifestyle as possible but I knew there would come a day when it would no longer be in my control.

After ONLY my very FIRST visit here, I felt more energetic, more optimistic, and more vibrant! I felt like I was walking taller, like things were brighter, my attitude had improved, and I was happier! EVERY subsequent appointment, I could feel things changing. I could SEE things changing! I was VERY DEFINITELY on the right track!!

In the week following my medication elimination, my skin was smoother, my gray hair was fading, my hair was smoother and more manageable, I was thinking more clearly, sleeping soundly through the night (no getting up throughout the night), my body measurements were changing, my clothes were fitting better, and I lost FOUR POUNDS (in ONE WEEK, WITHOUT trying!) I predict 2016 will be a GREAT YEAR for me AND my family BECAUSE of the care I have received at Baker Chiropractic!

I never realized what a difference a chiropractor could make! Before coming to Baker Chiropractic and Wellness, I thought all chiropractors were the same! I was never so happy to be wrong!!

Dr. Brock and his staff have all been so helpful. Without his dedicated staff, Dr. Brock could not focus on his patients and their care, as well. Everyone has their job, what they do best and the entire office operates like a well-oiled machine! Everyone has been so positive, patient, and informative. Baker Chiropractic and Wellness for ME has been a Godsend!

I want to thank EVERYONE involved in my care now and in the future!

— **Melissa N.**

• • • • •

At the end of 2011, Betty Higgins embarked on a unique journey with Baker Chiropractic and Wellness to lose weight and gain her health.

At 55 years of age, Betty had struggled with her weight for decades. That battle was taking a toll on her overall physical and mental health. She suffered from a long list of health conditions from fibromyalgia to depression to high cholesterol and was taking thirteen (13) different prescription medications to treat the symptoms of her various ailments. The list included such common prescription medications as:

- Lyrica
- Celebrex
- Lipitor

- Allegra
- Atenolol

Betty had tried all types of diets in the past including the ones that are highly advertised on television by celebrity spokespeople.

However, those diets failed her and left her frustrated. She needed something different. She found the difference when she stopped into the Red Bank Clinic of Baker Chiropractic one day and talked to Dr. Paul Baker.

"I felt a strong leading from the Lord just to stop in (the clinic) without an appointment", stated Betty. "They took me right into this bustling office, just liked I belonged there. The rest is history", she added.

Betty had a strong desire to change her health and her life, but she had not found the right program with the right support. Unlike the highly publicized diet plans, Dr. Paul's and Dr. Patrick's LifeCall Weight Loss and Health Gain program is not focused solely on weight loss. In fact, loss of weight is simply a derivative of their unique program.

A LifeCall is about making changes to your lifestyle in order to gain health and lose the elements in your life that are preventing you from having good health.

When Betty started her LifeCall program in 2011, this is what she said about why she was doing it:

"I would like to be able to take better care of my grandchildren. I haven't mentioned it to my daughter, but the reason I won't take both grandchildren outside to play together my myself is that I'm afraid a four year old and a two year old will outrun me and I couldn't keep them safe. I'm ashamed to say that, but it's true. I came to Cincinnati from a failed marriage which in part was caused by my obesity. I would like to regain my health and my life."

In November 2011, Betty sat down with Dr. Paul Baker and Dr. Patrick Baker to discuss her LifeCall program. They provided her with detailed plan to escape her unhealthy habits and develop a new and healthier way of life.

The doctors showed Betty how to eat, taught her the importance of proper nutrition, provided her with guidance on exercise and set a schedule of regular chiropractic care with Dr. Paul.

Betty's first steps in her LifeCall program began by throwing out all the processed foods in her refrigerator and pantry that were providing her with little or no nutrition. Then, she went on a special shopping tour at a local supermarket where she was showed what food to buy and what to look for on the labels. The doctors also gave her a detailed exercise plan to follow along with regular chiropractic care.

For the last twelve months, Betty has been following the LifeCall program, attending routine chiropractic care with Dr. Paul and enjoying the support and motivation of the Baker Chiropractic and Wellness staff. Her investment in herself is paying huge dividends. Here's what Betty has accomplished:

- Lost 70 lbs. of weight.
- Reduced dependency on prescription medications from 13 to 3.
- Self esteem restored.
- Confidence increased.
- Positive outlook on the future.

"If someone would have told me I would be 70lbs. lighter in one year, I would not have believed them", said an overjoyed Betty Higgins. "I had tried to lose weight and keep it off for 30 years and had lost hope until Dr. Paul's and Dr. Patrick's LifeCall program", she exclaimed.

Betty is an inspiration to anyone who is facing weight and health conditions. Her determination and hard work are providing her with a new outlook on her life. She is a perfect example of how strong faith and support from others are essential to conquer adversity and promote positive changes.

· · · · ·

My name is Ken Rice. I am a 62 yr old man that had never had chiropractic care.

In 2009 I had a total hip replacement which was the result of osteoarthritis. At this time I was given a prescription of Meloxican for the arthritis. Six months later I started having pain in my neck. I went to my primary care and he referred me to a spine surgeon. I was sent for a cat scan with dye. The result came back that I would need to have a procedure to put cadaver bones in my neck due to the osteoarthritis. After praying about my situation I decided to hold off on the surgery, at which time they recommended I stay on the Meloxican. I was also on blood pressure meds and had been for quite some time. I am a local beekeeper in Fairfield, Ohio. In the summer of 2012 it was time to extract honey.

I was out on one of the farms pulling boxes off the hives that were full of honey. Each box weighs approx. 65-70 lbs. I must have turned the wrong way and a pain shot across my lower back and down my left leg. I thought I strained something and with some rest, it would be ok. The pain didn't go away. So I went to my primary care physician. They took x-rays and sent me to a neurosurgeon. He said I had a herniated disc, and we would try epidural injections. I went thru a series of those with little or no results. All the time remaining in almost unbearable pain. I couldn't stand walk or lie down without the pain. I was desperate for some relief and I didn't know where to turn.

A wonderful friend that goes to our church (Geneva Lewis) begged me to go see Dr. Patrick Baker. This was approx. 2 months after I had injured my back. I made the appointment. The day of the appointment I could barely walk in the office. I was slumped over and the pain was obvious on my face. Dr Bakers staff greeted me and took me right back and did x-rays and scanned my back. The scan showed my neck and left lower back were severe. I waited in the Dr's office and Dr. walked in and said Mr. Rice, We are going to help you. They had me hang over a machine as long as I could. He adjusted me and when I got up off that table I was standing straight and my pain was decreased by 40%. I could not believe what one visit did for my pain. With every visit my back continued to improve until I was pain free. We are still working on my neck, which was more severe than my back. I have so much confidence in Dr Baker and his amazing staff that I know we will get my neck pain free also.

My wife Carol and I took a 30 day challenge that the Fairfield office offered. It was literally a life changing experience for us. We were to use recipes from the Maximized Living nutritional plans, a book offered at Dr Patrick Baker's office. We weighed in on a machine that told your weight, body fat percentage, and muscle mass. After the weigh in, we started our 30 day challenge. The recipes in the book I will have to say are absolutely delicious. We started every morning with a protein shake which was a scoop of Maximized Living Protein powder. That is added to 1 cup of almond milk. To that I would add fresh Kale, fresh strawberries, fresh pineapple, a few almonds. The book is a wealth of knowledge for nutritional values on various things. For example, you would need to eat 20 bowls of oatmeal to equal the nutritional value of I bowl of Kale. I put the fresh kale in the protein shake and when you blend it up you don't even taste the kale. After a couple weeks we realized this was a life style change we could live with. We both work, so what makes it nice is any of the recipes can be done in 20 minutes or less. The recipes literally explode with flavor. After 30 days we weighed in. I lost 14.2 lbs. and reduced my body fat by 2.8%.

My wife did even better reducing her body fat by 3.6%. An added amazing fact is that both my wife and I are off all prescription meds. Including blood pressure, arthritis meds, acid reflux meds, and cholesterol meds, just as a side note. The acid reflux was caused by the extended use of arthritis medications. It is now 61/2 weeks and I am down 20lbs. and my wife Carol is doing well. We monitor our blood pressure every morning just to keep tabs. So far both are at or slightly below normal with no meds.

We are at a point in our lives that we are living a much healthier life because of the total program Dr. Patrick baker and his amazing staff offer for everyone. It's not a diet. It's keeping your spine in alignment and discovering a nutritional plan you can follow and enjoy the rest of your life.

I thank God for directing our path to Dr. Patrick Baker and his staff. Dr. Baker and his staff truly care about a person's quality of life. My wife and I are living proof.

God Bless.

— Ken R.

• • • • •

90
Whiplash

I recently went to Baker Chiropractic after having a fall where I hit the back of my head. I was having about four different symptoms that I first had checked out by my doctor. I passed the typical office neurologic test, so he sent me home and said I was fine! The symptoms continued so I decided to go see Dr. Brock Frear.

After the initial visit and exam, I saw where I actually had a form of whiplash that severely affected my C1, C4, and C5. I also had other areas of my spine that were off and needed help, but not necessarily related to the fall. The great news was that it was all reversible!

Once my corrections are mad my spinal nervous system will be in working order again and my body will be healing itself properly again. I learned the spinal nervous system must stay free of spinal stress when there are subluxations in your spinal column then there is the cause of your spinal stress. All of my symptoms are all gone and I am so grateful to Dr. Brock and Baker Chiropractic!

— **Beth P.**

• • • • •

Other Books by Dr. Paul Baker
and Dr. Patrick Baker

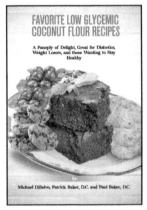

To request a copy of one or more of these books, please contact us by calling **(513)-561-2273** or send us a message from our website at **bakerchiropractic.org**

www.bakerchiropractic.org
(513) 561-2273

3 Cincinnati area clinics:
- 4781 Red Bank Road, Cincinnati
- 675 Deis Drive, Fairfield
- 7556 Voice of America Dr., West Chester

If you live outside the Cincinnati, Ohio area and would like to become a patient, please visit our website for travel information and special appointment scheduling.

Made in the USA
Middletown, DE
28 August 2023